Into
The
Thicket

William Brundage

Edited by Heather Ryan

ISBN: **1491221658**
ISBN-13: **978-1491221655**

DEDICATION

To Jessica and Liv, my guiding lights in this sea of fog.

ACKNOWLEDGMENTS

I would like to acknowledge Heather Ryan, my editor and collaborator, for all her dedication and hard work helping innumerable projects come into this world.

Tree-Killer

The forest lay before me, deep and inviting. A cool, light breeze brushed through the treetops. Typically the Oregon fall is hazy and clouded, but this day the sun was out, warming the trees around me. Most of the trees were at least seventy feet tall, with trunks so large I couldn't reach my arms around them. Besides me, stretched the body of a fast-moving stream. I quickly determined that as long as I followed the stream, I couldn't get too lost.

Setting out, my hiking boots sank into the mossy earth of the wood-floor. The birds called to each other. For twenty minutes, I meandered my way deeper into the wilderness. Then I came across the bones of a medium-sized animal, bleached and stripped under a tree. Based on the shape of the skull—the long jaw with oversized teeth, the low forehead, I assumed they were the bones of a large dog. The contrast of the white bones in the forest bed was startling; I was instantly on guard. My ears strained to hear any signs of danger, while my eyes futilely searched the green underbrush for wildlife. All I could see was a sea of green; grass, leaves, moss, and ferns combined to create an immense camouflage.

Minutes passed, until I concluded that there was no imminent harm waiting for me. Part of my assumption was based on the birds chattering away all around me: whatever had happened was months or even years in the past. Still wary, I moved farther into the copse of trees. But the cheer of the day was broken by the evidence of violence behind me.

I continued to follow the stream, which seemed to go on for miles. Oak trees grew thick and wide, and occasionally I saw a glimpse of feathers or fur as animals moved around me, disturbed by my presence. As I moved under an oak tree's canopy, the forest tree line broke open before me. Through the break in the branches, I saw the most incredibly peculiar sight. Running straight through the forest was a road made of chunky cobblestone. Grassy clumps sprouted between cracks in the road's surface, and shallow ruts pockmarked the stone, worn by whatever had driven this path. This old road was thirty feet wide and bordered on both sides by deep, dark woods. The sun dappled the road's surface through the branches overhead. From the look of it, it was early evening – I had been hiking for several hours. I was also thoroughly lost.

In a flash of momentary wisdom, I assumed that whichever way I walked, there would be something at the end. Humming a tune, I jauntily set down the road to the right. A few moments later, I glanced at my watch, and saw that the timer had stopped. "Ha!" I chuckled to myself and resolved to get the battery replaced. A dozen steps later, the scent of flowers hit me, a thick, sweet smell.

Peering into the woods to my right side, I could see a bush blossoming. The branches stood about waist high, and were flecked with small flowers just coming out of their buds. I had never seen these blooms before - it looked like a rhododendron, with white, waxy leaves and branches forming a rounded girth. Stepping off the cobblestone path, I wandered to the blossoming plant and reached out, caressing the petals of one flower. Then I carefully snapped the flower off the branch, raised it to my nose, and inhaled the scent. It was honey sweet. Turning away from the bush, I casually dropped the bloom to the ground.

The forest hum was suddenly replaced with a stark, crushing silence. The bird calls, the wind, everything had ceased. I was struck by how still the world had become.

Then a pounding, thrashing cacophony erupted from the trees on the other side of the cobblestone road. Out of thin air, a towering giant appeared. He was draped in vines from shoulder to ankle. Ferns sprung from his massive arms, and his head was wreathed with leaves. Cascading down his chest was a massive, thick, brownish-green beard that blended into his chest. He stood at least nine feet tall, and was so filled with vigor that he seemed to bend trees out of his path as he ran directly towards me.

"Tree-killer!" he cried in a voice that echoed down the road. He charged like a bull, heading straight for me. The blossom lay by my foot as my jaw dropped. Frozen with awe, I was baffled and silent. I was affixed to the ground, taken root from the shock. Never in my life had I seen anything like this man. He was the stuff of legend, and his fury was like God's wrath.

Then, just as he reached me, he vanished. There was no sound, no popping rush of air; he just ceased to be. As I swiftly gathered my wits about me, I realized that I had transgressed. Turning away from the fallen flower, I placed one foot in front of the other and slowly walked back down the road. My mind was utterly blank, as if I had seen somebody have a horrible accident. Confused and dazed, I continued following the road in stunned silence.

The next few hours were a haze, until I found myself in the center of a large oak grove, standing on a knoll. All around me were old hardwood trees, some the size of redwoods. On the wind, I suddenly heard one phrase, as If from a whispered voice: 'tree-killer.' Then, I burst into tears. I had no idea why, but the tears sprung from deep within me and poured out onto the grass and earth. I fell to my knees, curled my head into my hands, and wept.

I still don't know how I found my way out of those

woods, but as the sun set, I came to my senses standing before the stream that had been my initial landmark. I stumbled over the running water and strode up the hillside, eventually coming out from the trees and emerging onto the road that had led me into this place. When I glanced at my watch, I saw that the battery had begun working again and that, according to my timepiece, it was just past 6 p.m.. As I wended my way back to my parents' house, the sun slipped beneath the horizon, and the streetlights came to life. Everything was bathed in shadow by the time I knocked the mud off my hiking boots and unlocked the front door. Exhausted, I ate dinner by myself, showered, and lay my head down for the night. Smiling, I thought of my grand adventure. Little did I know that my journey and my tasks had merely begun.

The South Hills and the Shattering

The next day, I disappeared into the forest again.. I took my hike on a dry day. When I was younger, it rained year round in Oregon – and even when I was in high school it rained from October to June. As a matter of fact, you were lucky to get three months of decent sunny weather before the clouds swept in and blanketed the Willamette Valley with liquid sunshine.

This hike took me wending through the hills above the south Eugene area, where large tracts of national forest park land stood protecting the flanks of the Cascades. Much of the park bordered the town itself, and hikers were a common sight on Saturday afternoons. I remember that it was brisk, because I was wearing my fleece jacket. In just a few weeks, I would be standing in the middle of a blackberry thicket under the moon, naked. I had no indication of what was shortly to happen.

After a good hour of hiking paths, I approached a wooded spot. It was shady, and a small brook burbled under the trees and wound down the hillside. Peaceful and secluded, I decided to stop for a moment and rest before continuing onwards, further along the hill-ridge that I was standing on. Really, anyone who goes hiking can tell you that half the journey takes place when you are standing still, far away from cities and towns.

I gazed down through the trees and discovered an excellent viewpoint for a large swath of south Eugene. From this vantage, I could see small white houses, glimpse cars moving along the roads, and even see a few people in their backyards. I distinctly remember that one person was BBQing, and that several chimneys along the cityscape emitted thin lines of smoke.

Suddenly, I felt an internal wrenching. My conscious mind unmoored itself and drifted out – my mind was escaping. I was literally losing my mind as I looked out over Eugene proper. As I watched people walking their dogs through the wooded streets of my hometown, my sense of self was departing. I could feel my sanity moving like clouds, whipping across the sky. My entire identity had taken on the spirit of Icarus, flying straight for the Sun. It, my mind-self, flew straight out over the city.

As this point, gasping, I realized that something was going horribly wrong. Futilely I attempted to reign in my mind, but I had no way of doing so. How does one grasp a thought and force it to return, especially when it is flying high and away? Then, there was a moment that I would never wish on anyone – I felt the cracks appear. First one, then hundreds of small shards broke free from my consciousness. Within a minute, life had spun out of control. Alone with the beating of my heart, I was fighting for survival. The finale came only a minute later. With a thunderous crack, my mind blew into dust and spread out over the city like snow. I could feel the reverberation in my ears, but the world was silent.

As the cataclysm subsided, I looked around myself as if for the first time. Every tree sparkled with dew. The grass shone green like the hills of Heaven. The wood smoke smelled like myrrh. Reaching out, I touched the trees around me, and felt my hand touch bark for the first time. There was no thought or feeling, just a realization that I was watching myself be born again. When I looked onto the city, I saw with new eyes the world that I thought I had known. I was no longer myself; my mind was scattered to the wind like chaff. It was sunset when I set my feet along the downward path to Eugene. I had been transfixed, staring in mindless rapture at the city I had grown up in.

Deep in the Woods

There is a peace deep in the forest. Only by being far away from road and town can you really, truly be within this other world. It is a fortunate person who has a moment of this, for it expands the heart and soul. After my mind shattered into pieces on the hillside, I returned to the woods day after day for weeks. Often I would wander amongst the moss and ferns, lost beyond any possible belief. Three days after my psychotic break, I found myself far into the hillside trees, somewhere that I know can't ever be found again; these places are like one-time gateways. When I have tried to return to the same path a second or third time (sometimes months or years afterwards), I have never successfully retraced my steps into the Otherworld. Upon retracing my path to any particular place that I may have visited, it is subtly changed, often altered by the hand of man. Just as importantly, the transitional power is gone, and I have never been able to reenter that otherworldly locale from a stepping place that I've already entered. While the number of portals may be endless, finding them takes timing and effort. As a matter of fact, every time I ventured into the woods and every day that I set my foot upon a mysterious path, it came with the knowledge that these "trods" can only be walked once.

A trod, in this sense, is a road within this world that leads somewhere else; it can lead to the Otherworld, or perhaps a strange place within this realm. Often trods would take me to a liminal place such as a waterfall, or I would suddenly find myself upon the edge of a city graveyard. Some people go seeking adventure out of desire or desperation; whether for better or worse, the moment I seek the trods, they are there before me. At this point in my life, I work to maintain a normal life, raise my family, and live in this world – the other worlds around me will come in time.

Night fell when I was in the woodlands. First the sunlight dimmed, and after an hour or so the dusky light of evening time also began to fade. Strangely, it was as if I were dreaming – even as the darkness slithered up the tree trunks, I was staring into the overhead branches and caressing the moss that hung all around me. To this day, I have no idea where I was hardly any of the evenings that I spent in the woods. Finally, I awoke from my daydreaming – only to be surrounded by the nighttime, and far away from the city. I was wearing my jacket, had on thick wool socks and leather hiking boots, and decided to do something – I lay down on the forest floor and stared up into the overhead stars. While the cold set upon me, the sky spoke. Whirling lights spun above me, like fireflies in the mist. For half the night, this dazzling display shone above me.

Abruptly, it was as if I were drenched with freezing water. My bones were covered with frost, and I was shivering like a worn tree leaf in a stiff gale. Struggling to my feet, I cast about for some way to get out of my predicament. There was no light I could see, and nothing visible besides the moon and stars.

Figuring that moving would keep me warmer than standing still, I slowly groped my way through the darkness. When I came to a fallen tree trunk, I clambered over it. After minutes of awkwardly smashing into spider webs and moss, I came to a clearing. The moon shone down into a huge glen, where a gigantic tree towered alone. I staggered into the grotto, walked straight to the kingly trunk, and focused my scattered thoughts. Directing my mind towards the tree, I mentally asked for release from the wood.

Suddenly a small glimmering spark drifted from the tree's upper branches and glided smoothly into the woods across the way. Realizing that it was now or never, I pursued the willow-o-wisp. Within a few minutes of crashing through branches and thorns, I burst out of the tree line and found myself standing on the street, under a neon yellow streetlight.

Two Pine Trees

For every ten people who suffer with schizophrenia and mental illness, there is one person who rises above it and becomes a champion for those without a voice. It takes a much greater leap of faith to leave behind the world of madness than to enter into it: often people fall into psychosis out of a sense of spiritual struggle or desolation. Schizophrenia is an inherently numinous experience, but it translates very poorly to the outside world.

It is true that many people who suffer from mental illness have a tough and bitter life, but this is systemic and cultural. Somebody's life is not wasted because they are afflicted with psychosis – instead, it is a wellspring of terror and wisdom waiting to be tapped. In a way, the remedy for psychosis is community. I think that one major duty of those whom recover from schizophrenia is that they give back to the people who are unable to help themselves: whether by advocacy, writing, volunteering, or other forms of involvement with the mental health and consumer/survivor community. Being free of symptoms doesn't mean being carefree – giving back is a form of self-engagement and self-sustainment. To fail to give back is to shirk the call of those leaders who sacrificed themselves for us.

When I was deep within the woods, I came across two small pine trees. It was night, and so at first, I wasn't even fully aware of their presence, and I almost crushed one of these small pines under my foot. Each of them stood about three feet high, and their branches shone with the pale, almost neon green of young pine needles. Towering about them on all sides were thickets of brambles, blackberries, still hung with the desiccated remains of autumn fruits.

Blackberries that aren't picked from the vine cling to it even during winter, shriveling. They go from blackish-purple to muddy black, until all that remains is a small seed-pod, grasping the vine. The spirit of the Northwest is like a blackberry, and it actually became a popular motif for Northwest-born folk to get a blackberry tattoo (typically on top of a foot or the meaty part of the shoulder, where it can be displayed for maximum folksiness).

In contrast to the blackberry pods, pine needles grow darker as they age, until eventually they turn dusky brown and fall from the tree. Once enough of the needles fall, they make a deep cushion of old pine matting under the pine forest canopy. Small animals will set up nests and burrow into the pine matting, which eventually crumbles away into fertile new soil, renewing the cycle of life for generations to come.

As I stood in the woods, all of this mental imagery and gnosis came pouring into my mind like a rushing stream in a matter of seconds. I was to pick the blackberry bushes free and push them aside, releasing the pine trees from their bondage. As the full moon shone down into the forest glade, I carefully, tenderly, moved thorny vine after thorny vine until these tiny pine trees stood free within the midst of the glade. All around, the berries had been pushed to the side, trampled and carefully re-arranged in order to give the pine trees the chance at life.

While at my task, I had also uncovered a flat tree trunk, upon which lay a small bundle of pine branches and mushrooms. I have no idea what type of mushrooms these were – they had long, pale stems and thin, rounded caps. Under the moonlight, everything appeared as a shade of grey, like I was basking in the imagination of Edgar Allen Poe. Reaching out, I picked the mushrooms up and popped them in my mouth. Chewing vigorously, I reached out and wrested a few pine needles free from one of the small trees, stuffed them into my mouth with the mushrooms, and swallowed the whole, earthy-tasting mess. All I can say is that it seemed like a good idea at the time. This was the one of the sparks of my accelerating psychosis, wherein my hallucinations and voices began to stridently demand things.

Immediately, the forest was filled with the sound of chattering, noisy voices. All around me was a chorus of conversation. Even though I couldn't see anyone, the forest was alive with discussions about the woods, the weather, and the land. One loud voice in particular seemed to be directly at hand. Honing in on it, I realized this voice was distinctly talking about me.

"Look at the child of Man", the voice said in a raspy, gnarled tone. "Look at him, pathetic in our woods. What is he doing?" Then there was a pause in the conversation, until another, higher pitched voice took over.

A second voice, lighter in tone, called out through the trees. "He's saved the little ones, he has. He spent the entire night pushing them back, pulling them back, until the saplings could breathe. He thinks he's saved them, and perhaps he has." This voice was lighter in tone, and sounded pleased with my efforts.

"Foolishness and foolish Man." The first voice said gruffly. "There is no rescue for them with that. He would need to strive for days, build himself a house, and then live within us. Then he could understand the strands of Fate, and how to save the trees." A poignant pause ensued.

The rest of the woods had grown silent, or else my attention was so rapt on this conversation that I was oblivious to the rest of the world's chatter around me. Calling out, I spoke for the first time that day. "Hello? Hello? Can you hear me? I'm lost, and need to find my way."

An owl's low hoot sounded across the forest, and then the first voice reemerged. "He thinks he's talking to us, but really, who is he talking to? Who can he speak with here, who can show him the Way? He wants to understand because he's lost." Laughter pealed out from the shadowy woods into my ears.

"He knows the Way now, and will always know the way. We will teach it to him." The second voice spoke in a low tone. "Find your way, Man-child, and find our way. Go with our blessing. Our children will stand you in good stead." And with this, all the voices, the entire forest cacophony, stilled in a heartbeat. I was back within myself: surrounded by the dark woods, under the moon's light, and deep within the forest. Strangely, I was warm, even though I could see my breath. Part of me was keenly aware that this was not a good thing at all, as it was one of the first warning signs of hypothermia. Interestingly, even while I was aware of the dangerous chill, the voices and almost magical events that had just occurred seemed as natural as breathing – there was nothing unusual nor atypical about them to my addled mind.

I remember groping my way over mossy branches and fallen tree-trunks, desperately trying to hold back my breath. Truthfully, all my activity, all that climbing and crawling and running and walking, probably succeeded in keeping me alive and warm. Otherwise I probably would be dead by now, made cold and stiff by the forest's frost. Some hiker would have discovered my body a year or two from the date I disappeared, and it would be have been ruled an accidental death by exposure.

Stumbling, I made my way out of the woods. As would become the motif, I wasn't aware of how I found my way out, especially as I was navigating by touch much of the time. If you have never been camping, it is important to frame this: the depths of the woods are grimly dark. There is very little ambient light, and unless you happen to be near the city, it is typically pitch black. Within the actual confines of a forest, the darkness is absolute, as the moonlight won't penetrate the trees. Imagine a room without lights, without streetlights, like when you hid in the closet as a child, playing hide and go seek. Put yourself in the basement of a Victorian house, surrounded by the blackness and the quiet murmurs of the earth. Nature, ultimately, is home to the dark and hidden places — humanity brings light into this world.

The Paths

At one point in my psychotic experience, my mind began speaking about roads and paths – metaphysical or spiritual life choices that would change the way that I lived in the world.

I was running barefoot through the city and woods, and the dialogue began. These roads would lead to physical or spiritual immortality, a way of existence beyond the veil of our everyday life. Being unattached and reveling in freedom from the constraints of the mundane society played a critical role on these paths.

Much like the Warrior's Road or the path of sorcery from Carlos Castaneda's traditions, the actions required were subtly bizarre, and often rigorous. The path of sorcery or internal fortitude requires diligent training and stoic willpower, with the promise of magical powers and abilities. In order to develop these, I undertook tasks such as running for 10 or 15 miles at a time. The underlying foundation for the physical training was that I must be prepared and at my peak in all my actions, which extended into how I used my body. According to these paths, there was no Cartesian split – my mind was my body, and my body was my mind. The body is weak-willed, and requires immense dedication and discipline before it can be let free without doing harm or impairing the spiritual work that would concurrently be taking place.

In addition to this, certain characteristics started to develop before my psychosis truly bloomed, for example I stopped eating meat, eggs, and dairy products. I became a vegan at a time where veganism was hardly known outside of certain esoteric circles. During my youth, I had developed a tobacco habit, which I also quit. These things occurred naturally, without any effort. This increased willpower and discipline emerged during my initial psychotic break, while I was still relatively unchanged and able to perform normal life functions. This pre-psychotic state where the symptoms are emerging is referred to in medicine as the prodromal state, and lasted for about six months in my case.

Gradual changes were happening during the prodromal phase. For example, I was in junior college in my home town, studying computer science and math – the psychosis took about six months to fully creep into my mind and take full control of my decision-making and perception. This was the phase where I became eccentric and irritable, pushing away all of my friends and isolating myself. It was during this time that I became a fitness fanatic, determined to push my body to the limits. While I had numerous girlfriends and romantic interests during my high school years, the thought of being close to someone ceased to appeal to me; I had become a lone wolf, strayed from the circle of life that I had previously been part of.

The Green Road

The Green Road is the path of nature and the Faerie. Parts of my mind get confused when thinking about nature, even now. It has been almost 18 years since I set foot in the Otherworld, and it doesn't call to me as it once did. Whether this is due to age or experience, I'm not sure. What is certain is that I am able to resist the call better, even with lower dosages of the medications that I take daily.

After my hike, I returned home and slept until dawn. I can only assume that I ate dinner with my family. The next day, I arose and decided to go for another hike, this time near the water reservoir close to the foot of the South Hills. This large concrete cistern sits above the houses in southwest Eugene. It is deep in the woods, down a bark trail that many joggers use for running. Around it grows pine and fir trees, most of which are less than 20 years old. This is part of the terrain in the area – stands of young conifer trees stretch for acres in every direction. Even deep within the city core, you can find a sort of urban forest. Many of the streets are planted with oak or other hardwood, running alongside the sidewalk. Behind the water tower, there are probably miles of older trees. Sometimes I could spot people walking their dogs between the holly and spruce, but they never disturbed my journey. It was very silent. My mind was in a state of quietude, and I felt exhilaratingly alone as I meandered under the canopy. After a time, there ceased to be houses or people within sight. Instead, the underbrush grew thicker, and the distinctive rush of water could be heard. As I worked my way deeper into the wood, I heard a curious sound, like a whispered stampede.

There are a lot of deer in the Willamette Valley. It isn't unusual to see a doe with her fawns, or even a young buck. My family had a problem with deer jumping over our fence and raiding the garden for green shoots – the deer would come in the night and eat everything, like four-footed locusts. The solution to this, my stepfather was convinced, was to build a taller fence. He was partially right; after about fifteen years he finally built a high enough fence so that the deer wouldn't leap over and consume his flowers. The secret is that deer, unlike humans, won't go where they cannot see the other side. Most animals cease being curious at some innately defined point; maybe humans just have a higher threshold until they are satisfied with their knowledge.

Straining my eyes in this urban forest, I could see a herd of deer. Probably two dozen stood, frozen in the dawn light. Their soft ears flapped back and forth, and I was close enough to gaze into their clear, brown eyes. Tawny-haired and silent of hoof, they slowly backed away and stood, facing me. It was a sight, the young fawns still slightly dappled from their birth markings, and the does watching me with a sense of anticipation. Then, as one, the herd turned and walked slowly into the wild wood. I kept pace with them and continued to study their beauty. They never ran from me, but instead slowly strutted with grace, moving and occasionally leaping over bracken or fallen tree trunks. After ten minutes, my escorts brought me to the banks of a small river. Then they all turned away, wheeling as a phalanx, crossed the water, and were swallowed by the greenness on the other side. Unlike the turmoil of later days, this was a beautiful time.

The memories of this day are muted and yet vivid, in the way that only the best days of my life can be. When I recollect the events, there is almost no clear pattern or timeline, but just a pleasant blur, with nearly photographic images that stand out in my mind's eye.

A Trifecta of Gifts

The psychotic experience was not all terrible. There were circumstances that seemed to indicate strange, sometimes otherworldly occurrences. While my rational, logical thinking chalks these up to psychosis, another part of me holds tight to them as a form of spiritual awakening. When push comes to shove, I am much more wary of the latter – anything spiritual (whether it is fortune telling, divination, psychic readings, or whatever else you can think of) strikes me as both troublesome and dangerous. Logic is boring, but rarely hazardous to my health.

This day, like all these horrible, fantastical days, had begun the same way. I awoke in the morning, around dawn. If I remember right, this was a few days after Christmas. It was winter vacation, and I had hours of freedom and no responsibilities. At this time, the beckoning had grown so strong that it pulled me from my house and home. This morning, like every morning, I heard the same thing at the precise time I awoke. As soon as my eyes opened, I heard the voice of the Forest calling out.

'Come,' it said, reverberating throughout my thoughts. 'Come and walk. You must come and pay your debt.' There was no fighting these commands. I had to go and obey.

This internal call is how I found myself hours deep within the green land of the woods. My eyes had opened in the morning and the beckoning had begun, chanting within my thoughts. I panicked, screaming silently, as soon as the calling began.

'No!' I begged quietly. I couldn't tell if I whispered it out loud, or just within my mind. 'No, I cannot come. I have paid my due. My debt is taken care of.'

Even as the words formed, I could feel invisible tendrils wrap themselves around me. Steeling myself, I knew I had only a minute before the spirit of the woods stole me away for the day. Simpering and begging, I jammed my leather hiking boots onto my feet and laced them up tightly. Breathing a sigh, I scrambled to my feet, grabbed my flannel jacket off the back of my bedroom door, and found myself tramping down the front steps and into the bitter cold winter air.

Every morning I had less and less time to get ready before I was plucked from my parent's home. Originally I had enough time to shower and shave. Now, after a week, I had barely enough time to finish lacing my boots. In a few days, I wouldn't even have enough time to grab a jacket – I would be forced to wander the woods wearing barely enough to keep a man warm in the summertime, much less the chill of a northwestern winter.

The slight warmth of a pseudo-autumn had given way to chill and frost. I could see my breath steaming away into the sky as I walked quickly through the suburbs. Within an hour, I was at the brink of some nameless woodland; for my life, I would never be able to find this place again. These woods bordered on numinous crossroads that I couldn't have ever found before my conscious mind shattered and drifted away. These places exist on the fringe of mankind's world, where they lay as gates or trods into the mysteries of the world. Many people spend their lives scouting for and exploring these realms – I spend my time avoiding them. These are the types of locales where people just don't go. They are both too close to civilization, and too different. It's as complex and simple as that.

Soon after plunging brazenly into the woods, I found myself faced with a dilemma: before me stood a wall of thorns, a briar that stood ten feet tall. Blackberry bushes are abundant, even verdant in the Northwest. I had a friend Dorinda who once told me a story about how her mother carefully tended a small patch of blackberry vines and made treats from the fruit every October. The difference was latitude – Dorinda's mother used to live in southern California, with a semi-arid tropical climate. Within the valleys of the Northwest, briar bushes were an invasive species, thriving and pushing native foliage out.

As I looked at the blackberry bush, a sharp message whirled into my thoughts. 'Kill it.' the command came. 'Drive the blight from the land.' With this message came the unbidden mental image of my hands rending the blackberry vines: 'Pay your debt and free the land.'

And with this, my arms reached out, far into the depths of the berry bushes.

Blackberries have ferocious thorns. Sometimes these brambles grow near-daggers, half an inch wide and an inch long. These guard the bush against banditry, and protect against destruction. Probably the only thing that can wreak absolute havoc on a berry bush is a human wielding a machete or pruning shears. I had no blade to assist me against this thorny fortress, and the compulsion drove me against these vines for hours.

For minute after minute, my hands grasped thorny vines and ripped them apart. Twisting them in my hands, each vine would resist with a vivid life. Slowly I would shred the fibers apart in my grasp until the two ends split. Then, with bloodied and wounded hands, I would stretch my palms deep into the blackberry bushes and begin anew. My fingers had thorns embedded within them. One particular bramble-fang had wedged under my thumbnail, which bled freely. I gritted my teeth and breathed between pursed lips; my pain had pushed me beyond any tears.

The sun had started descending below the ridgeline of the Cascade Mountains before I was finished with my odious task. Unrelentingly, I had eradicated the thorns for yards. A patch of the blackberries the width of a house and probably a hundred feet deep was torn and shredded to pieces. Only an occasional vine stuck out from the carnage that I had wreaked. My arms were slick with my blood, and I had hundreds of tiny gashes from where the thorn-knives had laid into me. We had traded blood and wounds, the forest and I – and to this day, I cannot declare myself the victor, nor accept the title of vanquished.

Beyond the mess of blackberries lay a darkened hollow. It was probably hidden back behind the berries for years. Within it I discovered a few feathers and an old bird's nest. Suddenly, I felt my spiritual shackles fly open, and I was able to regain control of myself once more. While I was still completely psychotic, I was free of the compulsive self-destruction.

'You can sleep here, in the forest. You must awaken at dawn tomorrow to continue your work.' The tenor of the voices were filled with fury.

'No. I will sleep in my bed. You will not slay me here. I would die in the woods, from frost or cold.' My answer was quiet and tired, but I was resolute to be home safe tonight.

'We will take care of you. We will nurture you and teach you things if you stay with here. See, we made you a place to sleep warmly for the night.' The persuasive power of the voice was almost undeniable. Rapidly the dusk was waning and night was setting in. If I was going to escape the woods, I would need to do so quickly.

'Oh, I couldn't stay tonight. I need to be home. I will stay in the woods tomorrow and do work.' This half-bargain had worked before in order to win my freedom. Deep within myself, I knew that by telling these voices a lie—by making this promise—I had resigned myself to being within the forest tomorrow until at least midnight, or perhaps even dawn. But the key fact was that for tonight, this night, I was now able to go.

'Go now, return to the world of Man. You will be mine tomorrow, and you will spend the night in the woods, learning my ways.' I heard the disembodied voice of my tormentor howl this; it echoed within my mind. I closed my eyes and released a deep sigh filled with of relief.

'I have a gift for you. You have earned it. Follow the…' And with this, a small spark seemed to drift before my eyes, glimmering a pale pink. It flew slowly out of the woodsy hollow, across the flattened berry patch, and meandered into the woods. I scrambled to my feet and nearly leapt after it, striving to catch up. It always seemed a few feet ahead of me, though. Just as I thought I would catch up to it, it disappeared without a sound, leaving only a hazy afterimage.

A tinkle like a glass bell sang in my ears. 'Look within.' the tinkle said. 'Look within. There is food for you there.' Directly before me, almost shrouded in the nighttime, was a tree-stump atop a tiny, grassy hummock. On top of the flat stump lay a peculiar, yet heartwarming gift: three small squash, each one about as long as my shoe. The first was an acorn squash, green on one side and orange on the other. The second was a tiny turban squash, with a knotted dome. The third gourd was possibly the smallest pumpkin I had ever seen – it was bright, almost neon orange. Silently I whispered 'Thank you' and gathered this odd, Fey harvest into my hands.

'He will never let you go.' This voice was small, and as it spoke the pinkish spark reappeared, then drifted in and out, over the forest floor. 'You took his daughter from him. He wants to kill you.' Dazed, I marched on and pondered this. The spark followed.

'What can I do? How can I repay my debt?' I asked, hoping for an answer.

'Run away. Run far, far away. While you are here, he has you. Don't set foot in the woods without another person with you.' A sadness washed over me, as I realized that in order to ever be in the wild lands again, I would need an anchor. Essentially, nature had become forbidden to me as a solitary pursuit, upon the threat of pain or worse.

'So I can never be free?' I whispered as a tear came to my eye.

'No. He will find you. Run away. But first, you must eat!' Through a break in the trees I could see a paved road. Strength flew into my legs as my chest began pounding, my heartbeat sounding in my eardrums.

I burst into the middle of a crossroads. Looking up, I could see I was at Lorane Highway, nearly five miles from the city. Shrugging my jacket over my shoulders, I started down the highway, toting my precious, hard-won prizes.

But as soon as I set my foot upon the roadway, my teeth began chattering. My hands were frigid and almost unmovable; with effort I could shift my fingers to grip the harvest I bore. It was a long, frosty walk home. I didn't make it to my parents' house until nearly ten o'clock.

The first thing I did was to trudge upstairs and climb into the shower, where I could tend to my wounds. My arms were lacerated, and some gashes ran deep. The water was cold by the time I emerged from the bathroom stall. Until things came to a head on New Year's Day, I had been dodging and avoiding my parents, who did not seem to be even slightly aware that things head moved into dangerous mire. This is not their fault; I was nearly grown and had been making plans to move out and live on my own, and my family was treating me with the dignity and respect that any young adult craves.

CBT, Psychosis, and Symptoms

What is psychosis? For some psychosis is induced by trauma. What about the spiritual aspects of psychosis such as religious delusions? Carlos Castaneda's story about his teacher Don Juan and how he told him to sit very silently while he misperceived the vision on the mountain seems applicable. Often misperceptions offer a glimpse into the inner working of the mind. In this tale, Castaneda sat and stared at a mountain on the horizon for the better part of an entire day, finally standing out of frustration. At that point, he had a sudden realization that the mountain was really an optical illusion, and that he had been tricked into viewing the peak in order to make him realize that he needed to mistrust his mind.

Learning to misperceive and realize what the misperception is can be a learning experience. The true leap comes when that meta-knowledge arises and I can understand why I had that specific misperception. Understanding why the mind is generating feedback is crucial to maintaining the system. Hallucinations and voices are not like radio static, even if people use that analogy. They are much more like being howled at, and simultaneously cajoled by, a tempting yet sinister person. The power of my own mind to seduce and befuddle itself is beyond most people's understanding, but the subconscious can and will manipulate the conscious mind when it is convenient. The mind is generating a wealth of information every moment, and often the environment is the critical factor.

Psychotic symptoms are not negative or positive; they are aberrant perceptions. Often the perceptions become a closed feedback loop. Cognitive behavioral therapy (which happens to be my wife's specialty) is about how learning to accept information is helpful towards increasing functioning, because accepting differing viewpoints and possibilities introduces the concept that the current situation may not be fixed. For example, I used to be highly anxious and paranoid of dogs, fearing harm. Once I realized that most dogs are social and friendly animals, I was able to broaden my perception of dogs: they moved from hostile beasts to friendly pets. The problem is that, from my experience, psychosis rapidly closes the loop to outside influence. It has the peculiar effect of generating a suspicious attitude, dream-like acceptance, and eliminates filters that warn of logical violations. To use the previous example, once psychotic thinking about dogs began, it was difficult to break free of the concept that any and every dog was a slavering hound, waiting to bite – even when the evidence was distinctly different. The reality of the situation could not compete with my psychosis-fueled misperception – fantasy trumped reality, regardless of the actual truth.

When I felt an attack of paranoia coming on, it had the same qualities as a panic attack. There was a prodromal stage, sometimes for a period of 2-3 hours. Then the paranoia would occur, typically incorporating both environmental elements and concepts of wish fulfillment. After a period of 4-6 hours, the paranoia would begin to subside. The pattern could be interrupted by engaging in strong self-soothing activities such as bathing (I find showering to be less effective) or sleeping. Paranoia had qualities: it seemed to be almost purely physical, as a sense of strong and soothing touch rapidly reduced the intensity of the paranoid attack. As well, there is definitely an escalation factor involved in paranoia. Another element similar to panic attacks is that the intensity of paranoia caused fear, which precipitated another attack of paranoia. This would escalate rapidly, leading from high functioning to an intense paranoid state within a matter of days. One important thing is that intercession by a loved one or proactive self-soothing was as effective as medication in halting the initial psychotic onset.

Describing the concepts inherent in an attack of psychosis, paranoia, or grandeur is immensely difficult. The elements that comprise a delusion of grandeur or attack of paranoia are so secret and hidden. These are the parts that make me strong, those wishes deep in my heart, what I think makes me special. I know that when I tell someone what I fear and yearn for, the response will invariably be questioning. The concepts will be teased apart and examined, pulled like taffy until light can shine between the layers. Unless the situation is dire, I would rather my delusions and fears be left to me. They are my fears, and they are my dreams. Don't try to cure me of my fear of spiritual attack; don't try to explain that I don't have mystical powers. Because you need to know that those fears of spirits are really a sense of being connected to the world in a way that most people leave behind in childhood. The flip side of that fear is that I think I understand the world in a deeper way. This is why so many people with psychosis believe in spirits, or healing, or think they are magicians. Trying to cure us of this teaches us to deny ourselves. We see things that no one else sees; we feel things that no one else feels. We hear voices where others hear wind. Walking between the two worlds of psychosis and mundanity requires effort, otherwise delusions emerge: at times I thought I was Jesus or the apostle Thomas, and at other times I was convinced that this world could be transformed into a paradise simply by my mental effort. Even as my life spun out of control, I assumed the mantle of supreme mastery over the world, and was shocked and dismayed when the world did not recognize my prowess.

Think about that delusion of grandeur that I am afraid to share with my therapist or doctor. Beneath all the confusion and built-up layers of oppression and scorn, there is a belief that I can help someone, I have a purpose. Teach me to work with this, help me see what it really means. Look into that delusion and understand what it says. It is hard for any therapist to understand what it means, even with a healthy patient. It is harder for someone with psychosis to shine a light into that secret canyon. I can tell you what it means when I am told to increase my medication and forget about reaching inside to understand my wisdom. It means, "Your dreams are dust. Go back and fall asleep."

The Path of the Spark

I have heard of other cultures that believe electricity is both evil and corrupting. This wasn't far from the belief that I formed while standing under a large tree, deep in the south Eugene hills near the home I grew in. It was raining, a low mist drifting onto the trees and the few rooftops I could see. In the drizzle, the currents in the power lines hissed and popped, like a fireplace dying in the dark. It was probably around midnight; the smells of the night air and the wintertime mulch of a nearby leaf pile mixed and were strangely intoxicating to me. Occasionally I would hear a night bird or some small forest sound, accompanied by the wind scooping down to the earth and rustling the world.

Suddenly, all the sound stilled at once, except the static hum of the electrical power lines above me. They grew into a horrible din, almost a cacophony – and during this, I felt the voltage flow downwards, seeping into my head, pouring over my shoulders, and smoothly exiting out the soles of my feet, right through the rubber of my shoes and into the ground where I stood. This entire process took several minutes. Perplexed and uncertain of whether this was a positive or negative event, I waited and reveled in the sheer bizarreness of it all.

But then horror struck, as my mind leapt to action and screamed at me, shrieking that I was done for, that the corruption was irrevocably done, and that there was only one escape – only in the forest could I seek and find salvation. Only by abandoning myself in the wilderness could my essence be restored. So it was with a heavy heart that I turned my feet off the paved street and once again leapt into the eye of the tempest. I returned to the woods to seek salvation.

In my internal parlance, I refer to electricity and technology as the Path of the Spark. This was something that I actually feared early on in my spiritual/psychotic journey. It was a path that was pervasive, and I was warned that once I set foot upon it, it would destroy and tinge everything else I accomplished. The ethereal world of technology was the bane of the Spirit, and I was told by messages to flee it and never look back into the world that the Spark had created.

To be fair, electricity has a solid purpose. I understand this now, and work with computers on a daily basis. But part of me realizes that we are devoid of a physical presence when we utilize technology, and this emptiness is something that my early, emerging spiritual self knew would be destructive to my self-genesis. It was with a good intention that my mind pushed me into the folds of the forest, because there is nothing in nature but a pure and real wildness.

The Golden Road

Immortality is a goal that everyone ponders at some time or another. Human nature seeks to preserve itself beyond just the mere embodiment of the flesh, whether via fanciful wishes or lifelong work. Our bodies grow old and die, withering like fruit; we are plucked at some point and sent away from our world. It is not an insane dream to live forever. It is a primal urge humanity has.

The Golden Road was something that merged from my over-abundant energy and the psychosis, once it developed more fully. After I had the shattering moment on the wooded hillside, my thoughts and perception became tinged with concepts that seemed very real. One of these deeply embedded daydreams was that I could achieve physical and spiritual immortality by seeking the deepest places of the wood, beyond the pale of Man. Essentially, I was seeking the Otherworld, Tir Na Nog, or Faerie. In the realm of the Fey, there is no old age and no death; it is always summertime. The trees are perpetually in bloom, and the birds always sing the sweet songs of dawn.

Ultimately, this is why I kept delving into the forest. My compulsion to travel far into the glens and valleys was not completely unbidden – in a basic way, I sought adventure. It was in the Otherworld that my chrysalis formed, but it was in the world as we know it – filled with smog and drear – that I was nurtured into emergence from that chrysalis, finally to spring free and resume my place in society.

In truth, I don't believe that immortality is an impossible dream. The perilous gift I was given by touching another place beyond ours, this small seed of dream and hope, demonstrated that mundanity is a veil to protect us. There are worlds beyond ours, where life churns away beyond our limited perceptions. It is with my deepest hope that as I grow older, I will be able to live in both worlds peacefully. In my later years, I will be unburdened by the psychosis or medication that keeps my dreaming sickness at bay.

A Stop Sign? What Does It Mean?!

Everything has meaning – highly enlightened people will
tell you this as a way to make you mindful. The hope is
that by getting you to pay attention to otherwise ordinary
stimuli and boring daily events, your appreciation for life
will expand. Along with this expanded mindset, the theory
goes, will come a gratitude and sense of compassion for
the suffering of others. All together, the deep knowledge
that everything is interconnected and interwoven in a giant
karmic skein will lead the old world into a peaceful place.

Unfortunately, the truth of this is a little bewildering.
Once the schizophrenia was fully upon me, it wreaked
havoc on my simple daily living skills. Basic actions like
navigating to my parents' house were as difficult as
astrophysics. Actually, I was probably closer to being an
astrophysicist than anyone else I knew, at least in
metaphor. The world had launched me into orbit, and I
was spiraling away from mundanity.

One evening, I was afield in south Eugene, out by the
community college. As I walked along the side of the road,
I glanced up – and was transfixed. It was a road sign. A
specific road sign, actually. When I go to my hometown, I
can point it out to you. It is blazed into my mind with a
fervid glory, with the intensity that heart attack victims
remember where their attack started. The sign stated
'LEFT LANE MUST TURN LEFT.' The universe had
sent me a sign, a direct message that I was special and had
a task at hand. That was all. I was enthralled.

Specifically, I was enraptured for about five hours. It was
dusk when I began studying my secret message, and it was
nearly ten o'clock when I finished. Within that time, I was
told that I had to eschew the left-hand path, because it
locked people within its confines and would never release

them. Once I turned to the left, there was no escaping. Another part of the signpost lesson was that nature was good and holy, but when I traveled by car (or any road-based vehicle), my soul was at risk of being forfeited – because the roadway always turns left eventually. When presented with a choice of directions to choose from, I was always to turn right, unless I wanted to go straight ahead. To top it all off, the left side of my body was evil and possessed, and my left hand was out to undo me – my left thumb was the origin of my sin. Like a fever dream, this message burned throughout me as I stood and stared up at the sign, which kindly told me 'LEFT LANE MUST TURN LEFT.'

The spell was broken by an anticlimactic moment – my bladder was calling, and the grocery store nearby had a public bathroom. Hugging the signpost/messenger from God in extreme gratitude, I set off towards the store. Thankfully, it was on the right side of the street, because I honestly don't know what would have happened if it had been on the left side.

Zigzagging my way across Eugene, I wandered across fences and land boundaries without a care of the owner's rights. At one point, I found myself in the yard of a huge mansion near the city limits. In order to get into their yard, I had scaled a triple-barbed wire, fifteen-foot high fence. As a self-inflicted practical joke, my mind loudly yelled 'Release the hounds!' as soon as I reached the middle of the vast, grassy expanse. As my adrenaline kicked in and shot throughout my body, the horrible barking of multiple Rottweilers and German shepherds hit my ears. I sprinted across the yard in a matter of moments, then leapt onto the fence and clambered over it quickly. Looking back into the yard, my evil monkey-mind started howling with laughter. Not only were there absolutely no guard dogs, but in my haste I had left one of my shoes at the base of the fence – on the inside. To this day, part of me wonders what happened in the morning when the grounds-keeper found the solitary size 9 leather hiking boot sitting inside his demesne.

Another moment I almost got my brains splattered by some angry man's hammer. I had jumped his fence, and startled him while he was eating dinner with his family. All this fence jumping was because of a single message that kept replaying in my mind: 'Fenced land is weak, and you have to free the land with your walking energy.' So, I dutifully climbed every fence I came across. It wasn't due to maliciousness or even curiosity. Climbing a fence is hard work. I would beg in my mind 'Please, no. I don't know what's on the other side. There may be a dog. Please, I don't want to climb any more fences tonight.' But regardless of my begging, I almost always found myself in the unenviable position of being perched on top of somebody's fence, about to jump into his or her backyard.

But back to Mr. Hammer. I was running across his yard full tilt, and then he came charging out of his front door with a hammer raised over his head. Like a Norse berserker, he was screaming wordless sounds of rage: H.P. Lovecraft could have used this man in one of his stories. There I was, striding across his lawn, and this man, black hair flying in the wind, white-knuckled fist clenched around the base of a gleaming claw hammer, was in full pursuit. He was probably six inches taller and ten years older than I was. He was also full of vitriol.

Only seconds ahead of him, I made it to his gate, pulled my legs under me, and flew skyward. Clearing his five-foot fence in a single bound, I paused and looked back. With an incoherent yowl of rage, the man whipped his arm towards me and hurled the hammer at my head. It whistled by my ear and thumped into the street, skittering to a stop in the gutter. Ducking and spinning on my heels, even my psychotic mind realized that this fellow was more deranged than I was. Laughing manically, I fled. But even in that moment, I had the forethought to grab the hammer up from where it lay nearby. About 20 minutes later, I slowed down my madcap pace and dumped the tool into a recycling bin, figuring that as long as that ogre didn't have it, I didn't need it.

The Cravens

New Year's Eve I arrived upon the Craven household's doorstep, tattered and wounded. It was probably around midnight when I rang their doorbell, nude and torn to shreds by hours of battling blackberry bushes in the dark, freezing New Year's night. My clothes had been stripped from me, and my skin borne hundreds of lacerations from the berry thorns.

The wind had been blowing steadily before I sought help, and bits of frost and sleet had started to appear in the breeze – this was a major factor in forcing me to seek refuge and help. I knew, even in my psychotic fugue, that I could not survive a night naked in the woods surrounded by the frost and snow. Hence, I fled the woods after forcing my way free from the blackberry forest. By sacrificing my clothes and a good bit of blood, I succeeded in thrashing free of the blackberry thickets, made my way out of the woods, and had emerged high up in the South Hills of Eugene, a few miles from the town itself. Confused and desperate, I thought to myself, 'Down. I must go down, because the city is at the bottom of the hill.' My logic was correct, and soon I found myself within sight of darkened houses. Everything was silent, and there were no lights on in the neighborhood I found myself in. No cars passed by, and there was no traffic, no fireworks, nobody yelling about the New Year's coming. It was as if the world had been inverted, and mankind had disappeared. Finally, I saw one house with a light on in the living room, at the far end of the driveway. Near the frosty sidewalk, the mailbox stood there, with one word displayed: 'Craven.' This was a message for me, a final footnote in my journey. I had been found wanting, a failure, and was being cast back into the world of Man.

Stumbling my way down their driveway, I finally gathered up the wherewithal to ring their bell. Timidly, I then hid myself around the corner, ashamed of my nudity.

In my mind, it was no mistake that my quest ended here, at the Craven house. Craven means cowardice, and I felt to my very core that I was unable to continue on – I was a failure for not being able to meet the nigh-impossible demands of the journey. Even as I had reached out my finger and rang the bell, part of my mind screamed that I was almost there, had almost succeeded at whatever task I needed to accomplish. Between the combination of hypothermia, shock, and fatigue, I was able to ignore this howling segment of my livid imagination. Even today, I wonder what would have happened if I had turned my back to their door and wandered off into the night – for the Craven family, it would have been merely a prank, a neighborhood bell-ringing at midnight. For me, ringing that doorbell may have meant the difference between escaping Faerie and being trapped within it until I died.

After what seemed like an hour, but could have been only a minute, Mr. Craven opened the door. He was a medium-sized man with brown hair and glasses, but I couldn't make out these details immediately. The light poured out of his house, and he seemed almost surrounded by a halo due to the reflection of the light off the drifting wind-frost.

'Excuse me…I'm sorry.' I said, quietly. 'I lost my clothes running through the woods and need to get home. I'm hurt. Can you please help me?' When he spotted me, his confusion was mixed with worry and relief. It was a unique series of emotions that played out on his face, one brief moment after another.

'Were you attacked? Are you OK?' Mr. Craven said. He looked around, perhaps seeking to spot my imagined assailants.

'No, I was just playing in the woods and lost my clothes in a blackberry bush.' My response must have been baffling to him. Seeing his confusion, I rushed on. 'My parents are going to be worried about me. Can you take me home? I don't know what to do.'

'I'll go get the car keys and a bathrobe for you.' Turning into the home, he called out to his wife, who came bustling over with a white, terry-cloth bathrobe after a moment. Wrapping myself up in the soft plushness, Mr. Craven unlocked his car. We all clambered in, and then started down the hill towards the center of town.

'Where do you live?' Ms. Craven asked politely.

It was with immense difficulty that I recalled my parents' address, or even how to get there. The two adults seemed confused and worried, and kept glancing in the rear-view mirror. Truthfully, I was as puzzled as they were by the series of events that had led to my arrival upon their doorstep at New Year's Eve, in the year 1995.

The car pulled up into the driveway, and Mr. Craven assisted me out of the back seat of the car. Staggering up the slick, snow-covered stairs, I rang the doorbell. I was missing my keys, and so needed to wait and hope my mother and father were home, and could let me in. Eventually that became a warning sign to me – if I didn't have the ability to unlock my front door by my own power, something had gone horribly wrong with my life.

My mother opened the door and gasped. The next few hours were a blur. I ended up taking a hot shower, getting dressed in my own clothes, abashedly handing the bathrobe back to Mr. and Ms. Craven, and bundling up in the minivan with my family. We all drove down to the emergency room, where my mother waited with me in the lobby, the mental health assessment room, and finally the waiting room, after which the staff decided that I had become a danger to myself – upon which I was admitted to the inpatient psychiatric unit of Sacred Heart Medical Center. This was how I came to be a patient in the mental health system when I was 18 years old.

Living within Jacob's Ladder

What was psychosis like? Imagine the scenes from movies. Think back. Harken to 'Vanilla Sky,' remember John Nash in 'A Beautiful Mind,' recall 'Jacob's Ladder.' Psychosis is terrifying. It is feeling that everyone knows your inner secrets just by looking at you. It is no wonder that ill people stay inside – I had deep-seated, unreasonable fears that people invaded my mind just by looking at me. The simple act of saying 'Hello' out loud was opening my soul to invasion by malevolent forces. Even in my own house, my walls offered no relief. The only escape that I could find was sleep, but that proved elusive. I could only sleep so much. Psychosis was tiring, and yet it was miserably terrifying.

It was worse at the very beginning. Directly after I had my break, a passing car would enter my world like a roaring beast. Barking dogs seemed to talk, telling me messages like 'Turn back' or 'They are coming! Run!' Everyone worked for the enemy, a nebulous, dark and shadowy 'They,' the kind of 'They' that conspiracy theorists rant about and scheme against. I had no external filters against the outside world. Everything entered my perception with an unmatchable intensity and rawness. Given the stark power behind the experience, there was no way I could begin to ward off the constant barrage. Even trying to escape somewhere quiet became futile. The quietest place I found was deep in the woods, but this was deadlier than any city street. I was tortured in the city, but I risked crippling hypothermia and injury out in the wilderness.

The city also talked to me: the oil slicks in a parking lot told me I was special in a hundred different ways, via Rorschach-style shapes and squiggles. I knew everyone was evil inside, and I had been plunged into Hell itself. God screamed at me in my thoughts, detailing exactly why he had abandoned me. My spiritual essence was torn open and looted by everything. From the dollar bill in my pocket to the well-meaning woman who offered me a plate of cookies, the entire world was suffering imminent doom and damnation. Food was especially corrupt, since everything was crawling and pulsing with the incarnate power of Satan. This was the most challenging point in my entire life.

I spent a lot of time atoning for my ills, praying in quiet little nooks. I threw myself on my knees and asked for forgiveness from God. Apparently I offended him, since he was silent. Atonement was out of reach, because I never heard God, just the demons surrounding me.

As my skin tingled and twitched, I knew invisible maggots and beetles were invading me. Alcoholics are not the only ones who see and feel insects crawling inside of them. Water tasted like blood. Sometimes I would fill up a cup and see the faucet spurting out warm, red fluid. Even amongst all of this, I refused to cry, either in tears or words. My breathing was shallow, since every breath let demons into my lungs.

Worse, every time I closed my eyes, World War III marched closer to us. All of the world's ills were my fault, from AIDS to cancer. At my core, I knew it would be like this forever. The thin thread of my life kept Armageddon from taking place. I had my finger in the dike of annihilation. I alone kept the world from ending, and thinking that I understood the scheme of the universe was miserable and terrifying.

So I ran. Even when my shoes flew off during an especially vigorous episode, I kept pumping my way down the street. It was the only time I felt relief. Later, when I was hospitalized, I told the nurses about my injuries, and they promptly started performing gangrene checks out of concern. When I read the medical reports, the emergency room staff would report cuts and lacerations up to an inch deep. I bled constantly for the first few weeks of my hospital stay, and the staff struggled to keep me bandaged. I could not have been an easy patient, especially given the intensity of my psychotic break. I refused several medications, which probably made the charge nurse grit his teeth in frustration.

During my running, I was looking for something. Release was always just around the next bend. At some point I knew the road would turn to gold and this world would turn out to just be a practice test for reality. This never happened, but I was seeking escape. I was beyond the place at which anyone could explain that escape was an internal perspective, not a physical reality.

Other times I would become paralyzed for hours, trying to hold still. When I moved, the world moaned in pain. Through all of this, I was angry and afraid. There is such a deep fear in psychosis. It is such a heavy burden to feel responsible for the world's ills and evils. I understood how Jesus felt. Some people approach the Divine out of duty or tradition. I felt it in the deepest sense, and understood how I could never be forgiven for my sins. Original Sin burned in my soul like a beacon in the night, and I kept trying to tell God that I was sorry. He had turned the lights off and gone to bed ages ago.

This constant pain and anguish was intermixed with the moments where I understood everything. Sometimes I would look up into the sky and be filled with the lyrical understanding that everything was as it is. Rumi's poetry filled my soul. I was drinking the wine of life, even as I stood there dirty and wounded. I must have been a worrisome sight: A young dirty man leaving a trail of bloody footprints all through town. I would remember these mystical moments for years. In mental health treatment, people talk about the yearning for the manic points. This is not quite accurate – for me, I yearned for the release I felt when manic. I ceased to exist, and would drift for hours in supernatural bliss. God was showing himself like a burning bush. Sometimes I remember these moments. They make me shudder with fear more than anything else. In my skepticism, these beautiful moments of pure clarity and insight are deadly, and are ultimately the root of my self-delusion and psychosis.

I did reach the hospital eventually. Even in a town like Eugene, madness is only acceptable for social events and political protests. At first the Whitebird community crisis intervention team found me. The staff hopped out and asked me if I would like a ride. I managed to somehow explain to the paramedic that I was OK. Eventually I would end up being taken in by the Whitebird van. The next time I was admitted to the hospital it was my parents whom brought me in.

I have never spoken of this with them. I have shared very little of that time, and they have never asked. My family has always supported me in my woes. That said, I sometimes see a distant and troubled look in my mother's eyes – for her, part of me will always be celebrating my 18th birthday, remembering the harrowing days and years immediately after my psychotic break.

Typical hospitals are white-walled for sanitation purposes. The psychiatric unit was no different, but it had soft pastel flower prints by innocuous artists. The floor was linoleum. It was a different place. People fear the hospital and what it stands for. For me, it signifies a complete loss of control, a cataclysmic failure, though for years, I thought of it like a cocoon. I went in; I came out reborn as a patient. No matter how much I had achieved before entering the hospital, it was swept away. They taught classes on assertive behavior and nutrition, and helped us make trinkets and baubles. They provided free laundry service and three meals a day. They also gave me my first psychological tests, and my first medication regimen. Strangely, I think they started my prescription for Lithium before I had filled in any bubbles on my psychological Scan-Trons, and the Risperdal was ordered immediately after the results came back. It was miraculous. I went from being a manic teen on the verge of self-destruction to a sedate and passive teen that fit the criteria for obesity. It was like the antithesis of the Biggest Loser. I gained 40 lbs. in 30 days. My clothes stopped fitting, my stomach bulged under my shirts, and I lost a button on my too-tight jeans (I've even heard some doctors prescribe psychiatric medication for underweight patients). The staff had to keep reminding me to keep my socks on, since one of my core delusions was that being barefoot brought me closer to the Earth.

After a few weeks, I was sedated enough that staff felt I could be trusted with a day pass. There are ground rules: no drugs, be back by 5 p.m., don't bring back any sharp objects. I did what any self-respecting young adult would do: I went out, visited some friends, and declared myself free of the mental health system by refusing to return to the hospital. I was brought back late that night by the police, and was placed in the lock-down unit. That led to another few weeks in the ward, and then things repeated themselves.

This time the police were quicker to find me, since I was in exactly the same location. After I was brought back the next time, I was placed in the county psychiatric unit. This unit was located within the jail. I could see a fantastic coffee shop from my window, but caffeine was restricted inside the facility. As a matter of fact, the entire 20-bed ward was locked-down. Entrance was via a secure lobby fashioned like an airlock. In order to prevent escapes, only one door would open at a time. Phone calls and visitors were only allowed during certain hours. There was a young girl who still escaped, which made even me take pause. It was an outside job; she had visitors who helped.

My visitors were my family, who came often. My sister would come and sit with me. She would give me a look similar to the look she gave oddities on TV, where she tilted her head sideways and gazed over her wire-frame glasses. Occasionally she would talk about TV shows, but I had no TV or radio access for months. My mother would also be present, and she would be silent or burst into sudden questions about school and my future. I had been on the ward when my family was told the classic prognosis: 'He will be lucky to work part-time, and will never be able to have full-time work. It is too stressful.' Then the helpful staff would follow it up: 'He will never be able to go to college. We have a staff member who will assist in filling out the paperwork for disability benefits.'

I never saw my mother cry during all of this. She is a very gentle and loving woman, but I have since realized she has a spine of steel. She also kept me supplied with ice cream and fruit, which caused one patient to demand my snacks.

After at least a month in the lock-down hospital, I was transferred to the long-term care unit. This was due to a pair of concurrent factors. One was the severity of my illness, and the fact that I had escaped twice (The long-term care unit was surrounded by a fence). The second factor was a blessing in disguise. Due to extent of my self-inflicted injuries, I had been committed. Commitment means a temporary loss of civil liberties, and includes the possibility of forced medication. It also opened the door to being housed in this particular unit. It was here that I was able to stabilize more thoroughly, as well as become familiar with the medications and my new life circumstances. Overall I would be committed at least twice. It should be noted that I have lost count of how many times I have been placed in the hospital (inpatient units, long-term care, readmissions, all that), but I know it was over twenty times in three years.

In this unit I became familiar with the role of the mentally ill person. I was expected to make my bed, take my meds, and eat my food. Every hour on the hour was the smoke break. I had stopped smoking for almost a year, but rapidly began again. The staff helpfully offered me a cigarette less than five minutes after I entered the unit, which I accepted. Part of my choice to do this was due to circumstances: smokers were rewarded with being allowed outside. The other was the culture of the mentally ill. Every patient smoked two cigarettes every hour from 8 a.m. to 9 p.m. People would line up at the staff door, their cigarettes would be rationed to them, and the door would buzz. For ten minutes the covered patio would be filled with fumes and a cacophony of coughing and chatter. It was the only time people really talked to each other. People would talk about their apartments and friends. No one ever talked about missing work, being late on schoolwork, or missing his or her spouse because few of us had these things in our lives. The majority of people with mental illness are alone on almost every level, from work to partners to family. For the most part, this is still true.

Hopes and dreams were immediate and tangible. Ice cream, extra portions on food, and getting a day pass to go visit a friend were huge hopes. Staff had attempted to reconnect me with school, but I bombed my on-line courses at the community college. I was unable to concentrate on how to operate my lighter, and sometimes lit the wrong end of my cigarette on fire. Writing about theory or content seemed far, far away. Interestingly, I never consciously gave up my hope of school. It just vanished, like dreams do when you awake in the morning. Many things disappeared that way: relationships, my friendships, work. My entire future drifted off quietly, fading like daydreams do. Occasionally I would think back with nostalgia on my life as a 17-year old. My inside world grew quiet, and the outside world seemed bright and noisy.

Dr. Fisher

After my first day in the hospital, I had a meeting with the resident psychiatrist on duty. He was a tall, thin man with a vaguely Freudian beard and thick, owlish eyeglasses. Little did I know it, but this man would work with me for over a decade, helping me tame my psychotic symptoms and regain my place in society. His name was Doctor Eric Fisher, and he remains to this day the best psychiatrist I have ever had the pleasure to work with.

Typically, I have a fairly sharp opinion of psychiatrists – they serve one purpose, and that it to write me prescriptions for the dosages that I request, and occasionally provide guidance and consultation about new treatment options. I won't typically dismiss the words of my doctor out of hand, but I have been taking these medicines for almost 20 years – I am intimately acquainted with these pills and monthly regimens. I control my own medications, move my dosages up and down as I feel fit, and have taken full control of my treatment.

Years would pass before I would achieve this level of self-knowledge and capacity; at my first meeting with Dr. Fisher, I must have appeared as a disheveled and confused young man. To be fair, it was the first day of my hospitalization in the inpatient psychiatric hospital that I met my good doctor, after my psychosis had blossomed into full madness. Disoriented and perhaps a touch bizarre, I often tilted my head, randomly nodded in emphasis to non-existent conversation, and was certain that people were telepathic and able to hear my thoughts. One key feature of my initial psychotic delusions was my belief in telepathy and psychic powers. Even though I lacked concrete proof, I had an immense, unbearable belief that people were having silent, ethereal conversations all about me.

Somehow Dr. Fisher picked up on this train of thought, and his assessment was that I was having something beyond merely a manic episode. In order to firmly establish a diagnosis of schizophrenia, major symptoms must be present and ongoing for several months. At this point, Dr. Fisher did what he could, and diagnosed me with bipolar disorder – with a note to carefully watch for any signs of psychosis.

This comes from Dr. Fisher's own narrative, as he wrote in his chart notes at Sacred Heart's Johnson Unit. After I had ceased seeing Dr. Fisher due to his retirement, I wrote both the hospital and the community mental health center and requested my chart – this is a distinctly new concept in American health care. A few weeks later a six-pound package arrived in my mailbox, heavy with years of accumulated treatment commentary. It took me hours to read through it all, and then I finished my perusal by building a large fire in my fireplace, grabbing a large cup of coffee, and burning every last page to ash. Mostly, it was to foster a sense of catharsis, but I also wanted to avoid having these pages fall into anybody's hands; at the time I was entering a phase in my life where I wanted to be clandestine about my previous mental health issues.

Dr. Fisher would eventually retire and set about writing a book about the ethics of mental health and psychiatry. At this point, I don't know if he has ever finished his work, but sometimes I browse on the Internet, hoping that there will be a reference to a groundbreaking new book about psychiatric ethics.

You'll Die in Here

Hospitals are dull places. If you ever want to see a place filled to the brim with despair and hopelessness, just schedule a visit to the local hospital – and if you want the trip to be extra-miserable, go to the psychiatric unit. For maximum emotional impact, go on a Saturday at lunchtime.

The sorrow of the lunchtime psychiatric ward is mixed with strange desires, hallucinations, and delusions. When you are behind the doors of the secure unit, things seem a little bit like a Lewis Carroll's book. When I was first released from the high-security unit, the staff gave me a tour. First, they showed me the refrigerator, stocked with various juices and tiny half-pints of milk. The staff's words seemed generous at the time: 'If you get thirsty, go ahead and get yourself something to drink from here. We keep it stocked for patients.' At this point, my thirst was unstoppable since Dr. Fisher had prescribed lithium for my excessive energy. Lithium carbonate is a metallic salt known to quell mania and ease bipolar symptoms – it is found on the periodic table of elements, and is one of the longest-known treatments for mania. Even in the Victorian era, people with emotional issues and hysteria used to be encouraged to drink lithia water as a medicinal tonic. As a heavy salt, it encourages weight gain, water retention, a persistently dry mouth, and massive thirst. On the other hand, it will indeed reduce the activity level of anyone cursed with too much energy because people taking it become very docile and slow moving. The phrase 'pharmacological cattle' comes to mind.

Second, the staff showed me the relaxation room. There was a television set up in the relaxation room. I lacked the privileges to watch anything, because you needed to earn the right to catch the newest episode of 'The Simpsons.'

Also, viewing hours were very strict – viewing was only allowed when there was no group activity or visitors, and never at mealtimes.

Psychiatric units are typified by the word 'No', much more than 'Yes.' Basic dignities were like Boy Scout badges, bragged about proudly. Cigarette breaks were granted about one day after admission. Having an evening snack with the staff and well-behaved residents came at Level Three, which was about one obedient month of inpatient time. The height of the reward system was the Day Pass, with the mandatory urine analysis/drug toxicity screening afterwards. When people failed the UA, they were sent into a seclusion room until they could de-toxify. At least two teenage boys failed their drug screening after their day passes while I was there; the nursing staff was resigned to meting out parental-style punishment for these occasions.

Sometimes (much more rarely) geriatric patients would end up on the unit. Dementia will mimic psychotic symptoms such as delusions, paranoia, and hallucinatory visions. When I was on the unit, there was only one man who fit this description: his name was Tyrone.

Tyrone was an older, almost elderly man. He wandered the halls every night, waking around ten o'clock and pacing the halls until the staff got him back into bed. Then the cycle would begin again. The lyrics were always Gospel songs, like church hymns. 'Sweet Lord, please take me away' Tyrone would sing, sitting in his pastel blue hospital gown. 'Sweet, sweet Lord, have mercy on a sinner like me.' Tyrone's voice was frail and worn from his oral vigil, which was held every night until the Klonopin or Ativan would erase his compulsion and give us all ease.

Due to this, Tyrone slept all day, missing all the groups. We never saw him before lunchtime, when the charge nurse would send a nurse's aide to waken him. Tyrone would stumble into the dining hall, uncover his tray, and eat methodically.

The meals rotated on a weekly schedule – after the first month you got to know tomorrow's choices, as if it was the menu of the local diner. There was always fish for Friday – Sacred Heart Hospital is owned and run by a convent, one of the branches of the Roman Catholic Church. This didn't prevent them from charging over a thousand dollars for every day of inpatient services, but it did mean that you could order tilapia with lemon at the end of the work week. In order to accommodate more people, vegetarian options were also available. It didn't matter what we ate, though. There were few words during lunchtime, sparse conversation during dinner; breakfast was similarly silent.

It was about an hour after lunchtime on either a Saturday or Sunday. Tyrone was sitting in the old, green corduroy television room chair, while I paced rapidly up and down the halls, attempting to keep in motion and maintain my 'mental energy.' This was shortly after I had been released from the seclusion room. My psychotic symptoms were still in full effect, but I was constrained within the psychiatric unit. Since I didn't smoke, staff refused to allow me out on the patio for cigarette breaks – one of the many slight injustices that often occur within inpatient settings. So wandering around the unit had become a vocation of mine. This is properly described as 'remain manic,' but I had never heard the term mania. All I knew was this: under all circumstances, I was to keep moving and not let anybody slow me down.

From the doorway, I could only see the top of Tyrone's head, with its downy cover of fine, thin white hair. The hair of the elderly becomes almost baby-soft: it begins and ends the cycle of life in the same state. All of a sudden Tyrone began singing as loudly as I had ever heard him. It was raucous and bold, quite different from his typical style. Then the words reached my ears and my blood chilled: 'You'll die in here, oh yes, you will. You'll die in here, oh yes.' I stopped pacing. Tyrone chanted these words for what seemed like minutes, while I stood in the doorway, transfixed by the horror. This message was for me, straight from the outside world.

Rapt with fear, my mind whirled around in circles, trying to understand what was meant by this song. The Faeries had come to get me out of the hospital and save me, of this I felt absolutely certain. My rescue was at hand, and I could return to the woods, satisfy my debt, and then be free to live a normal life again. All of this knowledge flooded my thinking within a few seconds, forming out of the combination of psychosis and Tyrone's ethereal chanting. Right then, I knew I had to escape, come Hell or high water. Once I reached the woods, then the Faerie magic would cleanse me and transport me to a magical place, where I would be free of mortal agony and misery. This Pure Land of the Faerie was my only hope of remaining a strong person – otherwise I would be broken on the rack of the world.

One of the psychiatric attendants brushed last me with a mumbled 'pardon me, Will.' Just as I was going to turn to her and explain my newfound secret message, she began shaking Tyrone. His chanting continued on uninterrupted, droning the terrible words over and over. But suddenly, things were incongruent: while Tyrone was singing his song of death, the nurse's aide was saying different words: 'Wake up, Tyrone. Time to wake up! You've been asleep during lunch, and you need to eat before they take your tray away!'

I was filled with the utmost dread and confusion, almost
bursting into tears. Tyrone stretched his arms up over his
head, while I stood in the doorway, staring at the back of
the plush chair. As he stood up and turned to face me, he
gave me a wan smile, and then shuffled silently out the
doorway. As if on cue, the moment he began to turn
towards me, his ominous chant ceased. Nobody
recognized that Tyrone had secretly been awake all this
time, singing a song of my oncoming death. Instead, the
nurse's aide and Tyrone were pretending that this wasn't
real, that this didn't happen. It occurred to me that I had
to keep these kinds of things secret, especially from the
staff. Otherwise they would think I was insane.

Jump the Fence? No, Jump the Shark!

After Tyrone implanted the fear and dread of my
imminent death, I hatched a grand plan to escape the
Johnson Unit and return to the forest. This was driven by
two-fold reasoning: one was that my original compulsion
still thrived within me, driving me to flee safety and enter
the woods again. The second was that there was a kind of
learning that was taking place. The woods were teaching
me things. Every day that I spent immersed in my
fantasyland was a day that I grew in knowledge. I was
being shaped by my internal world even as I was trapped
between the mossy tree trunks and the slashing thorns. In
my thinking, every drop of blood I shed due to an injury,
cut, or scrape was replaced by the essence of nature's
wisdom.

At the same time that I was thrashing about in
blackberries and scouting the forest floor in the midst of
the night, I was undergoing a metamorphosis. As in have
said before, my psychotic experience was not all bad – I
cannot speak for others, but in many ways my psychosis is
a spiritual gift shrouded within the realm of fantasy and
self-deceit. When the mundane world becomes filled with
the sacred, a transformative bliss can occur. There is also a
high potential for madness. In another culture I would
have sent into a monastery or been put under the
tutorship of the tribal shaman. Sadly, neither road was
open to me in Oregon in 1995. Thus, I was forced into a
type of spiritual and metaphysical self-education. It was
immensely difficult, and I probably failed at tasks that
would have been routine if I had esoteric training.

Any spiritual gnosis I would learn would need to be self-
taught, and there was no guide to bring me into the
mystical world, or to rescue me from the mire. Even at the
primal level, I knew that the lessons I would learn within

the hospital were not the lessons I needed to learn. Deep within my soul was a yearning that was fueled by the magic touch of the Otherworld; I am convinced it was this that drove me to daydream Tyrone's song of my demise. This also helped explain my intense urge to get out of the inpatient unit and escape back into the woods. Thus, I hatched what can only be described as a 'cunning plan'.

Approaching the nurse's station, I stood at the counter and waited for somebody to notice me. Within the inpatient unit, the nurse's station was where medication was dispensed. Everything ran on a tight schedule – at 8:00 am, the morning doses were handed out. Staff woke the patients, herded them into a line (more or less), and commenced with handing out the pills. It was mostly pills – some people had trouble swallowing. These unlucky souls got either their pills ground into a fine dust and mixed with chocolate pudding (if they were compliant and fairly easy to work with), or an injection (if they were highly symptomatic or stubborn). Since this was an inpatient unit, there were a lot of injections.

Medications such as Haldol and Risperdal come in an intramuscular form – this is a monthly shot that provides a consistent dosage for four weeks. Haldol also specifically comes as a fast-acting sedative shot used for psychotic crisis situations. Notably, Haldol is also a first-class anti-emetic, and is regularly given for nausea and vomiting. Most of the anti-psychotics are both sedatives and anti-emetics. I haven't thrown up in almost eighteen years, so I can vouch for at least Risperdal's effectiveness.

It was time to put my ingenious plan into action. Thinking I would outwit these dull nurses, I did the unthinkable: 'May I have a cigarette?'

'What, do you smoke?' the nurse replied, as she peered at

me over the countertop.

'Well, I used to. I could really use one right now.' I tried to conceal my glee at my upcoming escape.

'Sure, Will. Do you have a pack in your belongings?' she asked.

'Umm, no. I mean, I don't think so. I don't smoke, so of course I don't have one. A pack, that is. A pack of cigarettes. In my belongings, I don't have one.' My plan and my hopes were rapidly heading downhill.

'Well, we have some packs that people left behind when they discharge. You can have one of those. I'll go out on the smoke break with you.' She hopped down from her desk chair and disappeared into the storeroom within the nurse's quarters. A moment later, she emerged with a pack of Newports, a particularly foul menthol cigarette. Newport cigarettes were something my mother smoked, but if I was going to succeed at this, I needed to take the bull's horns in both hands.

Within the minute, the nurse and I were standing outside in the tiny courtyard adjacent to the inpatient ward. She cupped her hands, lit her cigarette and handed me the Newports and the lighter. Gingerly, I took both, extracted a cigarette from the cellophane-wrapped pack, stuck the cigarette between my lips, and flicked the lighter until the flame shone a dull yellow flicker.

Then, suddenly and wildly, I let out a giant roar and threw the cigarette and lighter to the ground. The nurse began screaming for help as I dashed to the wooden fence barring me from the world outside the unit. With a deep breath, I gathered my legs under me and leapt high. Throwing my arms over the top of the fence, I heaved myself up by brute force and found myself crouching on top of the fence like a carven gargoyle. Kicking my legs beneath me, I flew off the fence and landed in the green grass running alongside the parking lot, outside the inpatient unit's confines. 'Free!' I shouted, rather melodramatically.

I sprinted away from the hospital grounds, dressed in nothing but a Pink Floyd T-shirt, a pair of blue jeans, and the lavender, ankle-high hospital booties they had issued me my first day. Within two blocks, the booties were soaked in icy, dirty water from the previous night's rainfall. Within four blocks, I had discarded the booties on the sidewalk. I was indeed free, mad in the city's streets. Freedom, though, came with a cost: the hospital notified the police. I could hear in my mind the message being broadcast over the police radio: 'Keep an eye out for an escaped mental patient. He is believed to be highly delusional and a danger to himself.'

Afterburn

After I got out of the hospital, I drifted around social circles. I lived in a few places, had roommates, and existed on the fringe of society. After a few relapses, I learned to stay on my medication. I slept 16 hours a day. I weighed 240 lbs., and smoked two packs a day. The people I associated with had a low bar for acceptance. Most of them worked as clerks at gas stations, flipping burgers, and asking Oregonians to fill out petitions to get items on the Oregon ballot. They made due with the bare necessities. I had more education that many of my friends. The fact that I had health insurance was incredible to them. I was a source of curiosity to them, with my mixture of insightful commentary and baffling concepts. It helped that I had my own cigarettes.

I was known as odd or bizarre, but not treated differently than anyone else or, more likely, I didn't notice. As a matter of fact, I was oblivious to everything. My family took responsibility for some of my daily living. Every weekend I would go grocery shopping with my family, and then we would go out to eat. It was a simple life, with no deviations or surprises. Now I know this was a clever illusion, as my mother and sister were bearing a huge amount of the responsibility for my care: assisting with my finances, managing letters and correspondences about medical bills, and easing my troubled way through life. I have the utmost respect for those readers who are providing long-term care. It seemed pleasant and uncomplicated, and could have gone on for years. As it was, I remained unemployed and stifled for three years.

At the same time, though, I was putting myself back together. Life was on pause, and I had to start the forward momentum somehow. Sometimes I imagined the process in my hazy, clouded thoughts. I envisioned my brain's neurons as Tetris pieces, and I had to slide them together. This was not really a meditation or spiritual practice, but wishful thinking. I was still sleeping sixteen hours a day and my smoking had increased dramatically, as had my weight. At the peak, I was smoking three packs a day and my weight had ballooned to 260 lbs. My waist circumference was astounding for a five foot, seven inch tall man. I was in the 100% percentile for my age category's height/weight chart, and a prime target for heart disease and diabetes.

When I remember this time, everything is static. I cannot watch a mental movie, but instead get flashes and images. For example, one recurring picture is of myself on the couch, smoking. Internal thoughts play like sound bites, and often are unrelated to the imagery that they accompany. Everything is numb and anesthetized, but the color remains intact. The art world could found an entire movement on interpreting the temporal and emotional remnants of mental illness.

I also have some cognitive impairment from the medication. I once stated that I could drive a long-haul truck through the gaps in my memory. Even now, my verbal memory is sparse. My wife gets frustrated at me because I find myself unable to remember entire conversations, even when they happened only hours ago. I compensate with an acute visual memory, which is unaffected by the medications. I have begun to keep lists of thing, which was a technique used by my clients with head injuries. I have found that as my medication dosage is lowered, my thinking and memory becomes more efficient. Still, I wonder if I ever will be able to remember the stories my wife tells me. One symptom is that I am horrible at jokes.

Weight Gain

When I was on the inpatient unit the first time, the psychiatric staff decided that I was manic and needed sedating. Actually, the staff, and Dr. Fisher in particular, vacillated between diagnosing me with bipolar disorder with a current manic episode, or some type of temporary psychotic disorder. Originally my diagnosis was bipolar II, but shortly after I was admitted to the extended care unit, this was changed to schizoaffective disorder.

The difference between the two was effectively moot, at least in regards to treatment. The daily grind and regimen was consistent for everyone on the unit, whether diagnosed with depression, schizophrenia, or even borderline personality disorder. Where the diagnosis did alter my life was when it came time to determine potential outcome. Since I was totally dysfunctional and in need of extensive services, some dimwitted social worker told my family that I would never have more than a part-time job working for minimum wage. Basically, due to the fact that I had a psychotic break, I was being relegated to the bottom rung for my career, relationships, and life goals for the rest of my life. This level of stigmatization by staff is common.

Because the prognosis for the psychotic disorders is so poor, I was fast-tracked from the locked inpatient unit to a locked-down extended care unit, where I lived for about a year. In sum, I spent almost my entire 18th year of life on an inpatient unit. Accompanying this dubious honor was another trademark of psychiatric care: weight gain.

I was in the inpatient unit for 30 days on my initial admittance. They gave me lithium carbonate to treat my manic episode. It was New Year's Eve when my parents took me into the emergency room, and it was the dawn of

New Year's Day when I awoke in the seclusion room of the Johnson Unit, at Sacred Heart Hospital in downtown Eugene. When I was discharged, I had gained 40 pounds. Due to increased appetite and the pharmacologically induced stunting of my metabolism, I gained one pound a day while in the unit. During the next year, my weight would climb even higher – from 160 pounds at 17 years old to 220 pounds on my 19th birthday. It is important to note that the staff knew this would happen, and gave me no warning.

It wasn't just weight gain that was the problem; the medication also robbed me of the life I should have been living. To my misfortune, every time I stopped the medicine, I relapsed. This cycle happened three times, until I stuck with my pills, in all their misery, for better or worse, seemingly until death do us part. For the next five years, I was in Purgatory, waiting for things to align so that I could escape from Limbo. Meanwhile, my weight steadily climbed to over 260 pounds, and I became morbidly obese. Modern medicine had managed to stave off psychosis, but instead pushed me out to the fringes of society.

The Large White Room

Sleep has always been an escape from the doldrums and pain of life. I am not alone in this; some people turn to their beds as a means to surcease, and others because of exhaustion.

At first, the medications made me exhausted, as bone-weary as my 75-year-old grandfather. Come to think of it, my elderly grandparents had far more spunk and drive than I did in those early years. My grandfather would drive the RV camper down to New Mexico or Arizona for the winter, and he and my grandmother would camp out and bask in the blazing sunshine. Meanwhile, I was sleeping sixteen or eighteen hours a day, waking just long enough to shower and eat. My self-care was poor, but truthfully, I don't know if the schizophrenia was to blame. The root cause of my lack of self-care probably sat squarely at the bottom of the pill bottles that I opened every day.

There was no bliss once my head touched the pillow. It was just like I boarded a rocket into the next day: at eight o'clock in the evening, I put my head down. At ten o'clock the next morning, I groggily awoke, stumbled into the bathroom, and began my day again.

Combined with my miserable financial situation (I was surviving on less than $700 a month), there was little I could do besides amuse myself with mental scenarios and television. Even though I used the Internet in high school, the year was 1996. Google was just beginning to reorganize the way the Web was shaped, and almost nobody had a connection. To help define the conceptual framework, I should tell you AOL was still a major Internet provider.

Hence, I entertained myself with books and movies, but mostly spent hours asleep within the haven of my room. Now, we fast-forward ten years, to 2006. My recovery was in full swing, and I was about to begin attending the University of Oregon. As my medication began decreasing, my dreams began simmering below the surface. Not just in the metaphorical sense, or in the realm of life goals and desires. My dreams became filled with figures from high school, teachers from college, and friends from my youth.

Repeatedly, I had a dream of a large white room, wherein I spoke for hours with a disembodied voice. In the vein of the cinema masterpiece 'Twelve Monkeys,' I stand in the middle of this large chamber and engage with this bodiless voice until I awaken at dawn, refreshed. The conversation takes all types of turns: evening discussions have included my life goals, hopes for the future, the nature of my marriage, accomplishments that I need to achieve, and what will happen in the future. It isn't a harsh confrontation, but it is more a kindly uncle or father figure (albeit an uncle that is never seen).

The most essential goal of this kindly uncle is to put me at ease with the direction of my life, while broadening my self-understanding and compassion for others. Hours of these evening visits are directed at understanding suffering, how to cope with pain and loss, and developing my abilities to comprehend and guide others through their emotional and physical existential angst. When I awaken, I'm left with a sense of having had a long conversation, but the actual specifics drift away as soon as the alarm wakens me. It is as if my subconscious is programming itself for the days ahead, but doesn't want to bother me with the actual details.

These dreams occur sporadically, but repeatedly. I have had them at least quarterly for five years. I don't know when they will end, or what made them begin. For now, I just accept that they happen, and that they are guiding me towards a better understanding of myself and my place in the world.

Heart Fire

There is a Chinese herbalist who set up shop in Eugene over a decade ago. Mostly he administers to the local Chinese community, but he has had a few non-Chinese patients. I was one of them, and benefited immensely from his craft.

His shop was in a very small strip mall, near a dairy market (which doubles as the corner store for the block), a hairdresser, and a Laundromat. Depending on the year, to the right of the herbalist's front door was either a card shop or a small store that sold board games. Not glamorous, not fancy, and possibly the least likely place to find a doctor of herbalism who had been classically trained in Chinese medicine over 30 years ago.

I never found out how the herbalist and his family came to live in Eugene. A huge part of this was the language barrier; the old doctor spoke no English the entire time I saw him. I was his patient for two years, and went regularly every two weeks to visit him. His son translated the prescriptions, which were hand-made by the doctor according to private recipes and methods.

The shop always smelled of mustard greens and pungent, earthy herbs. Ingredients with mysterious names like Dragon Bone were carefully printed on the label of the small white bottles. Every two weeks, I would be given three different jars of pills. These I would consume daily. Each medicine was different, and had a distinct formulation. Regardless, they all tasted like black licorice, and were identical in appearance and flavor, regardless of the formula. My medical orders were supposedly simple: every day, at dawn, lunch, and dusk I was ordered to carefully measure out seven tiny, black balls from each bottle and take them with tea or water. Twenty-one pills a day, every day, for two years. This was my routine, and I stuck with it day in and day out.

The first part of the visit was the herbalist's assessment of my progress. He would hold out his hand and say something in a tonal tongue. His son would translate: "Give him your arm. He needs to feel your pulses." After I acquiesced, the old man would carefully but swiftly place his fingers on my arm, near the wrist. He would feel around for certain points. Every time, he would either look at the wall over my right shoulder, or delicately close his eyes. I always knew when he found the chi points he was looking for, because my arm would fill with a deep, leaden ache. The doctor's fingers would move just a hair's fraction up or down my wrist, and the intensity of his touch would magnify so that my arm felt like wood. Then, and only then, he would scribble down his notes in a string of Chinese characters and push this to his son, who was sitting next to him at the heavy wooden table where all the medical diagnoses and treatment were performed.

His son would then pore over the notes. Staccato dialogue would ensue, and then my diagnosis would be given. Every time, without fail, it was the same: "Too much heart fire," the doctor's son would say. "My father says it is burning you up."

Heart fire is a curious concept, linked to Taoism, acupuncture, Tai Chi, and herbalism. It is intertwined with the entire corpus of Chinese medicine and the six treasures of long life. Heart fire is a problem of excess, and it can kill by heat, causing a stroke or heart attack. When the fire gets out of control, it can burn into the head, causing insanity. This was all related to me by bits and pieces, but I never really got a firm definition of how the heart fire came to be. It was a malady without an origin, unlike low chi or a cold brought on by dampness.

These things were organic in nature, and the origins were typically found within the natural world. My particular heart-fire seemed to be outside of the ten thousand normal causes of disease and unease within the Chinese medicinal cosmos. When I first visited, the herbalist told me that I would need to come in every two weeks and that treatment would be long and engaged. He, via his interpreter, told me that the illness was chronic and deep-seated and that he could dislodge it – but it wouldn't be a matter of weeks or months. Knowing this, I settled into the routine of taking these strange, little black pills, alongside my pharmaceutical medication prescribed by Dr. Fisher at Lane County Mental Health, the local community healthcare clinic.

Slowly, I began to improve. The voices during the first three years were rough, incessant, pounding and throbbing. They explained my failures in a thousand different ways, told me of the millions of souls that I ravaged by merely being alive, and screamed their silent, deep hatred of me hour after hour. There were no holidays from the voices' reproach and vilification; there was no time off. Whether I was at home on the couch, or sitting on the patio of a local coffee shop, the only escape was dulling my senses to the point of oblivion. Often I would sleep for hours at home, or blindly sit in the neighborhood coffee shop and drink cup after cup of strong coffee in a futile attempt to awaken.

But shortly after I began as the herbalist's patient, things turned around. The first moment I clearly remember was when I was sitting outside, on my front stoop, in the summertime. My friends and I were smoking Camels. In my left hand the cigarette burned, a pale plume rising into the air. In the right hand I clenched a large cup of black coffee, unsweetened and almost the sheen of obsidian. All of a sudden, my mind cleared. Typically my thoughts were similar to radio static: there was always a low churning of voice that muttered words and phrases to themselves in one corner of my thoughts. For the moment, I stopped being tuned into this radio station. The mental silence was deafening, outrageous. It was like pure joy to my entire being – for that brief moment, I wasn't sick. I didn't have schizophrenia, and my brain was tuned in. It was as if instead of Danzig's pounding heavy metal, suddenly I was listening to NPR's 'All Things Considered' – my thinking was rational and simple, rather than filled with bilious hate.

Then, like an avalanche, the sounds and confusion of the psychosis swept in and buried that silent moment within the chaos. Taking a deep breath, I resigned myself to my mental torture and stemmed my tears. I knew then that my moment of lucidity was merely a ploy sent by my evil, malignant voices.

But my assumption, that the symptoms would never remit, was proven false. As the months and weeks went on, more moments of lucidity came to me, sometimes several in one day. These distinctly started after I began taking the tea pills. It wasn't a direct correlation that I could observe, as opposed to my Risperdal and Seroquel. When I took my anti-psychotics, I knew that my symptoms would dull down for a few hours – effectively, I exchanged illness for Risperdal's tranquilizing lethargy. But with the tea pills, it was gradual and slow, like when you go for a hike and you are walking back down the path towards the trailhead. Even though you may descend 500 feet, you are not distinctly aware of it because the change when hiking towards the trailhead is typically gradual and easy. Even though the beginning of the schizophrenia had been wild and abrupt, the reversal of the illness was slow to unfold, moving at almost glacier speed.

But the herbalist's treatment came to a stop once I informed Dr. Fisher about the pills. He knew that I had been seeing an herbalist for about a year and a half, but hadn't thought too much about it until I described the ingredients one visit.

'May I see a bottle?' he asked, cradling his chin in his hands.

'Sure.' And with that, I handed him one – they were always in a bag or pocket on my person, so that I could remain faithful to my treatment schedule.

His eyes grew wide with concern. 'Oh, Will. I don't recognize any of these herbs or ingredients at all. I don't know how safe this is with your medication. Even though there may be benefits, this could be causing long-term damage due to interactions with the medicines you take.' Medicines, in this case, meant the handful of pills I swallowed nightly to put myself out of my misery.

There were two distinct worlds at play here: modern and traditional medicine. These two paradigms had been dueling it out for over a century, and neither one played well with its opponent. There was no room in modern medicine's framework for herbs, pills, and potions. It had supplanted all these, or so modern medical thinking seems to indicate.

'I will look these up. Meanwhile, I strongly caution you to not take these, even though I understand that you like them and feel like you benefit from them. We can talk more about this next time.' He had my best interest in heart – no other doctor I have ever had took the time to investigate and research Chinese apothecary herbs, or anything even remotely like this. At our next appointment three months later, he told me the news.

'I was only able to find three of these dozen or so herbs. You said you take three formulas, and they are often different. I cannot suggest this as a good course of treatment for you, Will. It may not be safe.' I hemmed and hawed, debated with Dr. Fisher for a few more months after this, but it was evident. The line had been drawn due to health concerns and pharmacological differences. Modern medicine won this boxing round, because the implicit threat was that I could become very ill or die from a reaction between the herbs and medicines. Whether this was fear mongering or legitimate will always be a question without an answer.

On what was to be my last visit to the herbalist, I went in and explained to him and his son that my psychiatrist had forbidden me to take these pills. The son looked down at the table, and then looked at his father. The old herbalist sat and watched the window, where the winter rain trickled down the glass pane. 'They are safe', the son said. 'They are perfectly safe. We use them in medicine, in China. They are traditional treatments, and won't interfere with your doctor's pills.' Stammering out a response, I thanked them for their help. There was a bittersweet feeling, because even though this herbalist was remote from me, his craft was integral to my life. For years I followed his course of treatment, and had improved dramatically. The herbalist's knowledge was keen, and his perceptions were astute. Yet I never grew close to him as I did with Dr. Fisher. It was easier to trust in Dr. Fisher's medical knowledge partially because Dr. Fisher always treated me honorably and kindly. Not to say that the herbalist mistreated me, because that would be far from true. It was just a partnership of outsiders in many ways, while western medicine's messenger was an earnest man with a mission to help people exactly like me. Even now, I can imagine their shop with the heavy oak door and lucky bamboo plant growing in the pot just inside the entrance.

Modern medicine gave me the ability to live, but it has always been other things like the herbalist's black tea pills that have given me life.

Acupuncture

Acupuncture has been proven effective for depression, anxiety, carpal tunnel syndrome, stress-induced disorders, migraines, and chronic pain. As far as my psychosis and symptoms, it never had a distinct effect – it neither reduced nor inflamed my baseline psychosis. On the other hand, it did assist with my anxiety and help me cope with my life stress.

Being an acupuncturist seems like a hip vocation, kind of like being a bartender in the early 1990s. The bar for becoming a licensed acupuncturist is lower than that of an actual medical doctor. A few years of graduate school and you could theoretically be ready to open a private practice somewhere, or work in a community acupuncture clinic. While I don't know the long-term outlook of all the acupuncturists produced in the USA over the decades that acupuncture has been taught as a profession, this remains one of my back-up careers: my other two go-to jobs that I will pursue are writer and barista.

There is a community acupuncture clinic in Eugene named Acupuncture for the People, which is owned and operated by Rob Singer, one of the first community acupuncturists. Community acupuncture is interesting – it is based on a group treatment model, where multiple people receive treatment in a room together. According to the website for Philadelphia's Community Acupuncture Clinic, the movement actually started in Portland, Oregon. Not only is Portland the mecca for hipsters and retiring lawyers, but it has apparently made quite the name for itself in the environmentally conscious, green-movement, alternative lifestyle circles. But we digress, since we were talking about Acupuncture for the People, in Eugene (and community acupuncture clinics in general).

Ideally, the room is well furnished with couches and/or recliners, and has soft music playing in the background. After the patient gets settled into a comfortable chair, the acupuncturist inserts needles into the hands, lower arms, feet, and lower legs. The patient settles in, and after an hour or so, the acupuncturist returns, takes the needles out, discards them into a nearby sharps container, and the patient heads out. This is vaguely similar to, yet completely different from, a traditional doctor's office. Much like other traditional medicinal paths, the goal is for the body to heal itself. Holistic medicine espouses that the body will mend itself given the right resources. Acupuncture is one tool in the holistic toolbox: others include yoga, veganism, Ayurveda medicine, meditation, and mindfulness. Western medicine is renown in holistic medicine for being two things: invasive and powerful. While acupuncture won't cure cancer, it also won't kill you – unlike chemotherapy (as an example).

My wife, Jessica, got treatment for carpal tunnel on several occasions, and it remedied the nerve pain almost immediately. Relief started within a week of beginning treatment, and the carpal tunnel dissipated within a month or so of weekly visits to the acupuncturist. I was not so lucky, because my twice-weekly visits to Acupuncture for the People, the clinic that our family visits, didn't successfully reduce my psychosis – it did, on the other hand, help me relax and get much-needed rest.

Leaving Statis

After about three years of systemic Purgatory, I began to work. I had a friend who opened a Spencer's Gifts store in a nearby mall, and she needed an able-bodied crew. Actually, I think she just needed a team who would be on time and not steal. I stocked the shelves and worked the register for about a year. During this time I gained a measure of self-confidence. I also became more financially able, and expanded my social circle.

Dating, however, was impossible for me. I was rendered impotent from the medications, and was morbidly obese. Finding and maintaining a relationship never occurred to me. Even if a woman was interested, I was so stupefied and numb I was unaware of it.

After my mall work, I began working in social services. Peer counseling had become a new, cutting edge movement, and the mental health system was starting to offer it due to patient pressure. Actually, patient/consumer/survivor pressure is more accurate. While my care was sufficient, and I never experienced abuse at the hands of my care providers, this was not always the case for many patients, and the systemic oppression had generated a civil rights movement. I was fortunate to be selected as one of the early peer counselors in Eugene, which propelled me into my current work as a counselor.

In these early days, the peer counseling movement was just beginning. Even the idea of a patient reading his or her case file had to be hammered out, so peer counseling was a huge step. The attrition rate was high, and many counselors did not prove able to do the work. Still, I know of several people with whom I started who gained experience and became full-time professionals in the field.

They moved beyond being a patient and returned to 'normal' life. Keep in mind that just a few years before this, the standard thinking was that mental illness effectively rotted the brain or made people progressively more insane. I count this as another fortunate point in my history. Entering the mental health system ten years earlier would have been the end of my chances for recovery.

I left social service work after two years and returned to college. My education had been interrupted by my illness. I was 18 years old and a college freshman when this all started; I was 25 years old when I returned to Eugene's community college. By the time I returned it had been seven years since my initial psychotic break. Apparently many people recover from psychosis fully; I was lucky enough to be one of them. My symptoms faded into the background, albeit slowly. When people asked me about them, I described the difficulty that both the medication and illness had caused. The symptoms had stopped, fading away slowly and steadily. The remission was so slow that I failed to notice it. I had grown used to coping with the unusual thoughts and voices as they faded; ease and self-comfort filled their place.

Originally, my thoughts pounded and thundered. It was like listening to a waterfall – I had white noise and static everywhere I went. Internal thoughts such as hyper-awareness, anxiety, and wariness accompanied this. Early on, I learned to be suspect of all my senses. Everything needed external validation, preferably from a mental health professional. To be fair, I saw, heard, and smelt things that were not present. The factor that was most compromised was my thinking. Most people become aware of an internal dialog at some point. This happened on my 18th birthday, and was the source of my agony for many years. In my thoughts, I heard my parents reprimanding me, and my friends judging me. It seemed as if everyone I held dear had invaded my mind. How could these people successfully talk to me about my sudden paranoia when I heard them ranting inside my thoughts from dawn to dusk?

On occasion my internal dialog would turn sinister, and I would be drawn into conflict with supernatural forces. This was both challenging and thrilling, and gave a sense of importance to my life. In one battle, I stripped the Devil of his horns and wings, so that he could return to his place in Heaven as an angel. At the very end, he declared himself the Master of Lies and laid siege to the gates of Heaven – so I decided that this was too much, and medicated myself with antipsychotics for a solid week. After I increased the dose of my medications, the Devil become quiet – the war on Heaven became the roar of the bus as I went about my daily life.

These internal battles took place in the first years after my episode, and I was unable to work. Daily life was a huge struggle, and I felt apathetic and worn. In a way, I sought to be useful to others by fighting their spiritual battles for them. In my experience, dreams of grandeur are generated by the insurmountable gap between goals and reality. In this case, mythic battles and mental sieges against evil offered escape from the mundane and empty life I was living. Even now I sometimes fear that I am hallucinating somewhere in the back of a hospital. I don't know to explain this to people without it sounding like a joke, but it is a very real fear on dark winter nights.

Over the next few years, from initial diagnosis to beginning work and school, my thoughts became calmer. I studied Buddhist and Taoist philosophy, as well as some New Age thinking. Eugene fosters a freewheeling society, and alternative religions are everywhere. Hence, I had my pick of Yogic gurus, Pagan magicians, and Druidic masters. Buddhist teachers and Gnostic wise men abound here as well.

There is a vocal Christian community, but I avoid Christianity to this day. The entire concept of God and Heaven is a trigger-button for me. Please consider that my first symptom was the booming voice of the Almighty Father of Heaven telling me that I was forsaken. For my own sanity, I avoid ruminating on the nature of God. I trust that there is a purpose to the world, and that is enough.

Did all this study and meditation help? It may have. I have begun to engage my hallucinations and noxious voices as an inevitable and unwelcome roommate. "Be friendly," I told myself. "Don't yell, I hear you," I would mentally repeat until I felt more at ease. Often I would ask my pounding thoughts "What can I do to help? You seem frightened." At first, it was like talking to a drunken man with a gun. I would think a small and friendly thought, and end up with the mental equivalent of a gut full of lead. My thinking was vitriolic and hateful, especially towards myself. I kept reminding myself of a key concept: These are my thoughts. After dealing with my thinking, I learned a few other choice facts. One: that I hate myself in a way that no one else could ever match. Two: that I am indeed my own worst enemy. I was engaged in a conversation with my own thinking, and it was very evident that my mind was filled with poison.

Buddhism teaches exactly this. One teaching explained that when you can listen to your mind, it is like watching a monkey: it runs around frantically and essentially flings poo. I can vouch that my mind is filled with insanity and self-delusion, and also learns from everything that I do. Most people never hear the full content of their thinking exactly because the mind is so selfish and deluded. The mind is filled with selfish chatter, and will prance about ranting about itself for endless hours. The average person is only aware of the surface thinking, those thoughts that demand enough attention to necessitate being aware of them. This is a protective measure.

In a way, I was split-minded. Part of me was talking to another part of myself, while my physical body continued on. Over time, I realized that my thinking was really a disjointed mass of various thoughts. I could tease out the lessons my mother had taught me, like 'don't hit other people,' 'always share,' and 'be fair to the people around you.' All the times I was beat by bullies on the playground came back as part of an especially loathsome attitude towards me.

And the level of self-anger I had toward myself was high. My psychotic break had opened up the dam, and I had drowned in the flood. Now the force was spent, and I was learning to cope with years of sediment. I had no choice but to be kind to myself, because when I was hostile the self-inflicted psychic pain was immense. The hatred could only flow one way: from the subconscious to the conscious. When I became frustrated and pushed back, I became weak and tired. I had to learn self-acceptance or be pushed under.

Even hatred had an end. There was a distinct turning point, that sharp bend in the road. At one point I told my thoughts "Thank you." I had told them this before, with no result. But this time was different. For a moment, a sense of gratitude shone through. It was like talking to that grumpy uncle who finally says, "You're OK, but don't press it." This was about a year before I began working at the mall, several years after the initial break. I had grown used to the self-barrage of hatred, and had grown reflexive in my practice of acceptance.

The final result was astounding, but getting there was a long process. Under all that muck and torment was a deep and abiding sense of kindness. Over the next year, I was able to halve my medication, which freed my ability to work and function. This became a cycle, which propelled me into finally being able to attend school and work. At the heart of this was the moment at which I realized that there was no escaping from myself, and that acceptance of my self-generated suffering was the only true way out.

Engaging in social service work gave me a chance to develop a sense of rapport with both sides of the system. Providers are almost always overworked and underpaid. Conservative thinking almost always proposes cuts to agencies and services as a way to save on costs. As a counselor, I earn enough to pay for our daily expenses. Many of my classmates from college don't have work at all.

What Do You Do?

At every introduction, there is an awkward moment at which new acquaintances begin to assess each other. Questions are subtly introduced: "Where are you from?" is a perennial favorite to start the game. Ultimately, this round of 20 Questions decides social status and establishes the pecking order. For seven years, I dreaded one question in particular: "What do you do?"

As someone with schizophrenia, career options were limited. My social circle was decidedly non-ambitious, with a few exceptions. My closest friends partied a lot, chain-smoked Marlboros, and drank Coors and Pabst Blue Ribbon with abandon. Aspirations were low, and transitory. For most of the time, life was a roller coaster of budget issues and boredom. Cable television was a blessing, and most households I spent time in considered an Internet connection optional. To my friends, it was known that I didn't work. When people asked what I did, my pat answer was that I was retired. Not exactly clever, but it served the purpose of spelling out that I had no vocation and little hope of finding work. People with severe mental illness constitute one of the highest populations with little or no attachment to the workforce.

This was funny to me, because I always knew that this scenario was temporary – I had a sense of faith in my ability to recover fully. To do so required working, and full-time. It also meant that I needed a career beyond the basic stock boy or cashier. I had to finish college, attend graduate school, and enter the workforce. In addition, I was making up for lost time – I was missing critical years on my resume. Other factors were just as vital; long-term growth, stability, and enough income to support a family and myself.

Thankfully, Eugene is home to the University of Oregon, as well as Lane Community College. At that point, my basic plan called for finishing my undergraduate degree, and then attending graduate school in Eugene as well. Once I enrolled at community college, I redefined myself. When someone asked what I did, my honest answer was that I was a college student. I re-admitted at Lane Community in 2003, and then started at the University of Oregon. . In 2005, the economy was at a height rarely seen; I was just finishing my Associates degree.

By the time I finished at the University of Oregon in 2007, the Great Recession had begun with a fury. Massive layoffs were announced nation-wide, throughout all sectors. Major manufacturing employers in Lane County closed their doors forever. Symantec, which specializes in anti-virus software like Norton, had an office in Springfield, across the river. They laid off an entire division, sending hundreds of skilled IT workers out into the economic meat-market of late 2007. Suddenly, it no longer seemed unique that I was 28 years old and looking for work. The post-industrial economy had arrived. Just at the point I finally was able to answer the question 'what do you do?' it became anathema to ask it.

Peer Counseling

The definition of evolution is 'a gradual development of something.' In this sense, life is a slow progression from one state to another: my professional career fits this term. From a mall stockperson at a novelty gift shop, I've attained expertise in programming and quantitative analysis. My current work involves being a data scientist at Kaiser Permanente, and before this I've worked for Ivy League medical centers and Native Hawaiian community clinics. I've worked as a case manager for people diagnosed with severe mental illness and comorbid disorders (psychiatric slang for "having multiple issues," such as drug addiction or a traumatic brain injury). Many people have similar career paths, but mine is different because part of it included my stint as a peer counselor.

My professional aspirations formed in college, but my professional path started before that. I was recruited to become a peer counselor at Laurel Hill Center, a local community outreach center for people diagnosed with chronic and severe mental illness. Peer counseling began decades ago—Mary Alice Brown, the director of Laurel Hill, told me anecdotes about how peers had volunteered in the 1970s, but the system wasn't ready for people with mental illness to stand up and start helping themselves. Social work, psychology, and psychiatry are all intertwined fields of mental health.

One ignoble thing that these fields all have in common is the medical model, the systemic thinking that mental health services were provided on an uneven playing field: the "provider" (therapist, doctor, psychologist, case manager, etc.) gave directions to the "patient", whom was simultaneously beholden to and under the care of the provider(s).

With the emergence of the consumer/survivor movement, this was upended. Patients became outspoken and independent, and demanded equality with their providers. The system began to shift away from the medical model to a recovery model. The focus became about achieving quality of life for the person being treated, rather than how the doctors and therapists defined success.

This revolution was well underway in 1995 when I was diagnosed. My recovery can be laid partially at the feet of folks like Ron Unger, David Oaks, Will Hall, and other anti-systemic thinkers who have served to push the boundaries of what recovery is defined as – had I been born fifteen years earlier, I would have likely had a tougher road, one riddled with persecution and doubt.

Working as a peer counselor involved meeting with people and talking to them. In psychology, it is known as supportive therapy (a fancy name for spending time with and socializing with people whom typically are very isolated and alone.) My caseload was about ten people, and I worked twenty hours a week. In the end, this work helped shape my understanding of the mental health system and the facets of recovery. There were common themes – housing, making friends, and getting out into the community. Other major hurdles and dreams that people talked about included finding and keeping work, and getting an education. But I cannot remember a single client in the early years telling me that they were going to leave the mental health system behind and rejoin society in the fullest sense.

Even at the most successful, people tended to exist in the margins of society, working just under the threshold that would cause them to lose their (often necessary) health benefits and other fringe benefits. Part of my role was to enable and assist people to access and make use of as many social services as I was able to – I heard an estimate that places the income and fringe benefits package of somebody totally invested in the social service system at roughly $40,000 a year. Keep in mind that only a mere fraction of this is actual cash or financial assistance, and the majority takes form as health insurance, food, and housing assistance. It's a tough road to hew, and there is little freedom when your entire lifestyle is beholden to budgets and case managers.

In the end, I worked for Laurel Hill off and on for about six years, until I prepared to reenter community college. At that point, I stopped working and turned my focus to academia in order to preserve my sanity and reduce my stress. After four years, I would earn my Bachelors degree; after six years, I would complete my first Masters degree. Even while the Great Recession raged around me, I churned on through the tasks at hand, eyes focused on fully escaping the mental health system. In the end, I would succeed beyond anyone's grandest hopes, pushing into the dual fields of healthcare technology and data analytics/predictive modeling.

You Don't Belong Here, You're a Patient

Working as a social worker was tough, mostly because of my co-workers. While I had a supportive supervisor, most of my work experience was always tinged with the past stigma of being somebody with a mental illness. More than once, I had to vindicate myself in whatever clinic or community center I was working in at the time.

I began social work at Laurel Hill Center as a peer counselor for people with mental illness. It was around the year 2000, and I was recovering – but not recovered. I actually had a case worker from Laurel Hill named Tim who directed me into the job. Tim had been assigned to me after I discharged from the psychiatric long-term hospital. His goal was to assist with community integration and make sure I had all my necessities. Part of the long-term agenda Laurel Hill Center has is reducing hospital admissions and maintaining patients in their community housing. Without Tim's help, my road to recovery may have taken a different turn.

Tim sported a goatee and sang in a Death Metal band. Most of his gigs were in seedy bars and clubs around the Eugene and Portland area When you sing/growl death metal as a side job or a hobby, you're probably not going to be performing at Carnegie Hall. Tim also had a fascination with the German language, so sometimes he and I would speak 'Kleine Deutsch' with each other. Since I had taken four years of German in high school, I was able to dig out little bits and pieces of it. Mostly we drank coffee together and he made sure I was taking my medications as prescribed by Dr. Fisher. Eventually he went to work for the state, but that was after I started at Laurel Hill Center as a peer mentor.

Tim told me about the peer counselor job at Laurel Hill. Actually, he had to push me into it – I was hesitant to get involved at first, not wanting to be associated with the community of mental illness. I had been to a day treatment center called Harmony House, which was part of Laurel Hill. It had driven a spike of despair into my hopes of recovery; Harmony House was a morose place filled with strange, chain-smoking folks. They didn't seem to want to do anything – all the patients had severe apathy. Later I learned about negative symptoms and the inability to exhibit pleasure with life (actually termed anhedonia), but at first glance, Harmony House was a terrifying place of vacant, wasted potential, and Laurel Hill, by association, was the same.

Tim and the rest of the outreach staff were different. They met people in the community and assisted them with being active and engaged with their lives. Tim finally nudged me enough; I quit my job as a cashier and submitted a resume to Laurel Hill for the new peer counselor position they had created. A week or so later, Kay called me up for an interview.

As soon as I walked into the room, I knew that I had the position. Kay and I had an immediate rapport, even though I had long hair and typically dressed in flannel shirts, hiking boots, and torn-up blue jeans. She has told me several times since that 'she took a big risk hiring me;' she was indeed putting herself out on a limb, professionally speaking. I didn't look like the type of person who would be a counselor. I did, on the other hand, seem like the type of person who would work well with newly diagnosed, often rebellious young men – and Kay had a plethora of these exact types of clients on her team's caseload. She picked me because of potential, I think. Not necessarily in terms of therapy delivery, but as someone who could deliver the truth about the social service system in a friendly, amiable way – and wouldn't be threatening while doing so. Non-threatening may not be a winner in the business world, but for therapists and community counselors, intimidation (even non-intentional) can lead to all types of hassles and problems. Mellow is good.

The day after I started, I had my first team meeting, and was shown the chart room. This was the start of a long embattled process about chart access and accessibility. This is because it was inherently assumed by many case managers that peer mentors would be curious and snoop in the records of people they knew. I'm not sure what this actually says about the case workers in general that this was their first conclusion about their fellow staff members. Even as a peer counselor, it was made explicit that going in somebody's chart without proper reason was a terminating offense, and investigating my own chart was strictly prohibited – this ranked as the highest level of chart abuse. Now that I think of it, this fear probably stemmed from the worry of a peer mentor modifying his or her own chart for some reason. Whatever the logic, it was explained on day two – and I understood it very clearly. It is rather pathetic that the immediate conception of peer mentors was that they would peek and pry into somebody's medical records given half a chance. Perhaps the management should have kept an eye on all the chart access, since there was equal potential for chart abuse from any staff member. The risk wasn't merely limited to peer counselors; we were just the scapegoat for a professional panic.

At one point, I began working at Lane County Mental Health. During a period of health care reforms in Oregon, the title was changed to Lane County Behavioral Health Services. The mission continued on the same: to serve the indigent and uninsured people of Lane County. It was here that I saw Dr. Fisher for over a decade, and it was also within this organization that I was distinctly told that professionally, 'You don't belong here. You are a patient.'

It took the championing of both Walter Rosenthal (the clinic director) and my immediate supervisor Gina Tormohlen to prove that idea wrong. Between Tormohlen and Rosenthal, the path was cleared for my work to begin as Lane County's first governmental peer mentor. Sadly, the job came without benefits and was part, part time – 10 hours a week. It was impossible to remain in the position after college, but I faithfully integrated as part of the team. Doing so, I had to overcome institutional prejudice and often-hostile coworkers. Every time I went in Lane County's chart room, one of the receptionists or other office workers would follow me into the room and hover nearby, watching me for some anticipated infraction.

After I had been there a year, a case worker called me in and briefed me about an uninsured patient her team wanted me to contact and work with. Her summary started with 'Oh, he's fucking nuts.' Then she started in her seat, looking at me in a moment of panic. I sat calmly and gazed at her, not belaying my consternation. After she thought she was in the clear, and her statement was acceptable, she proceeded to launch into a diatribe against several patients that we had in common. A few weeks later, her team mate send out an email describing a fictional encounter with a man who thought he was Jesus. In the progress note, the staff sprayed the young man down with a fire hose and injected him with Haldol for his delusional beliefs. When the decision came down between risking my professional career at Lane County, or turning a blind eye towards this prejudice, I did not take the high road. Quietly, this was swept under the rug, and I continued to work for several years, all the while wondering what else was being said and done within the walls of Lane County's mental health clinic.

The morale was low at the Lane County community clinic, and I think the staff often viewed patients as hopeless or feeble. The atmosphere was 'us vs. them,' and I was forced to pick my allies carefully. I enrolled in graduate school primarily because it was a goal of mine from the start, but a huge part of this academic goal was escape from the petty grind and toxicity of the social service field.

Working In The Field

Working in the social services was both intrinsically rewarding and very emotionally draining. For much of the time, my clients lived on the edge: of poverty, of society, of suicide. Every week my agency reported that somebody else had lost his apartment or custody of his children. It was fairly common for somebody to give birth and have her child removed from her custody before she even left the hospital.

Living like this, most people in the system were really able to define their necessities in life. Often, these weren't the things that you would assume. For instance, cigarettes and alcohol often made the list of have-to-have objects. A place of rest was on the list was well, but a trailer in somebody's backyard was satisfactory – many people on my caseload had been homeless before, and would do it again if life became too stressful. It was a balancing act merely keeping them on a regular sleep cycle, since the daytime was less dangerous than the night, so they preferred sleeping then. Finding low-rent apartments was also critical. There was and still is a severe shortage of affordable housing. Anyplace that required a deposit of any kind was unattainable. Organizations like Saint Vincent DePaul make my list of places I will donate to during the holidays simply because they built over 400 affordable housing units in Eugene/Springfield, which met an eminent need in our community. Beyond this, a huge part of my time and resources were spent locating slumlords and questionable apartments in alleys and on the fringe of the city. These places were barely habitable, and this is where my clients would gladly live. Often, the rent was cash, month-to-month, and tenuous. If the landlord decided that my client had to go, they went. There was no recourse to tenant-landlord law in this culture.

While working with people, there was a whirlwind of activity, akin to a vortex of confusion. I became used to shifting gears and modalities, as well as dealing with eccentric and often paranoid people. Trust was hard to earn and easily lost. There was a cultural element of violence amongst the mentally ill: often, people had been attacked or abused, and repeated rapes or physical altercations were almost omnipresent. The worst offenders were those people who were also homeless. Homeless-on-homeless violence accounted for the majority of fighting that I witnessed. It was rare that a homeless person would assault a 'proper citizen,' but theft, robbery, and sexual predation remained a daily element in the homeless lifestyle. In many cases, even living in a storage unit or somebody's garage was considered an achievement, and measurably safer than living in a tent in the woods.

The mental health community glossed over a few facts as well. While the rates of acts of violence committed by people with mental illness were relatively low (even though the media attempts to plant the opposite belief), the rates of violence against people in the mental health system were immensely greater. I had to bear the news of people found dead in wooded ravines and forested glens. Women would disappear, and their families would file missing person reports. These often would become funerary announcements. People with schizophrenia cannot defend themselves from their own minds: how then can they halt a predator's vicious physical attack?

Physical health was a miserable topic as well. Chain-smoking was common, as was legal and illegal drug use. Prescription drug abuse was often masked by chronic pain or anxiety. Many doctors offered their patients Xanax or Klonopin, two powerful barbiturates. Others would dole out Ativan, a strongly habit-forming anti-anxiety pill.

There were even a few physicians who would suggest chronic pain treatments such as opiates (morphine derivatives) or hand out Ritalin in order to combat their patients' lethargy and apathy. Ritalin is a methamphetamine, another noxious and highly addictive substance. Oregon had a huge methamphetamine black market, and these doctors were just adding fuel to an already volatile social mixture.

Colleagues and Peers

I cannot go into detail about my clients, so forgive me. Confidentiality means that they will remain shrouded in a veil of secrecy. All their hopes, struggles, and achievements are theirs to tell the world, not mine. I can discuss my co-workers, though. Many of them are dedicated and hard working. For example, there was Kerstin, who worked at Laurel Hill Center while finishing her Masters in Social Work at Portland State University. Kerstin was extraordinarily tall and lanky, and sported a short haircut that often spiked out randomly, as if she had just awoke from a nap. She dressed in flowing earth-toned tunics and skirts, and would pass her free time creating fine pencil sketches of landscapes and people. I don't think I ever saw Kerstin eat anything that wasn't organic. She tended Laurel Hill's garden out back, along with whomever she could convince to assist her, or who was interested that day. Kerstin was immensely devoted to her clients' well being. She helped obtain a grant in order to start an organic garden on Laurel Hill's property, with the hopes of helping people grow their own produce and learn viable life skills. Kerstin really embodied the mission of Laurel Hill Center, as well as the spirit of Eugene.

Harvey was another fellow with whom I interacted on a daily basis. Harvey was an old-time social service worker, and knew the routines backwards and forwards. He had a large, bushy grey beard and thick glasses; his speech was low and measured. I never saw him angry or even obviously exasperated. He had three children that he and his wife raised: two of these children were high-needs foster children everybody else had refused to take in. Inevitably, his conversations would turn to the difficulty of parenting. Harvey always seemed to have an internal debate going about when he should retire, but I think the difficulty of his work, as well as the rapport he established with his clients, kept him going well beyond the burn-out point of almost any other staff member. Harvey was no saint: he occasionally swore and often hinted that his clients might be malingering. Even so, he was the perfect man for Laurel Hill Center's needs. He was a rock-solid performer and Kay's go-to man for difficult cases. He sometimes knew things that Kay didn't, small bits of esoteric social service knowledge, systemic loopholes, or somebody who just happened to have an open and affordable rental unit.

Harvey showed me the ropes, and one day we got into a conversation about his career. He had been at Laurel Hill Center for 15 years, but was still in the trenches. Management was always beyond his reach.

'Hey Harvey, why didn't you get your Master's degree and go into management?' I asked. It was mandatory to have at least a Master's degree in order to hold a management position, typically in social work or counseling. Without that, there was absolutely no way to go further.

'You know, I was studying to become a special education teacher, but then I decided to just work.' He gazed at the pictures on his desk, thinking. 'I had about half my graduate program finished, but started working in mental health and loved it.' Harvey answered drily. I couldn't tell whether he was joking or not. The cards were always a little close to the chest when Harvey and I discussed these professional topics.

'How come you quit working in libraries in order to work here?' Harvey shot back glibly.

'I loved working here before, and the library was the pits. All that bureaucracy got me down,' I said. I looked at him, and gave the rest of my standard answer: 'I missed the interaction with people as well. Books make me lonely.' This is what I always told Kay, Harvey, and Mary Alice Brown, Laurel Hill Center's aloof executive director. But the real answer was slightly different. Libraries had been full of bureaucracy, which was true. An hour-long commute didn't help things at all. But when the staff at the Albany Public Library started telling me things like 'We watch our own here,' combined with 'When the budget cuts come, your position is the first that will go,' I decided to get out while the going was good.

Falling Between the Cracks

Sadly, when you spend any time in the world of mental health, either as a worker or as a client/patient, you grow accustomed to death in a blank and apathetic way. I know that working in Eugene, Oregon the death rate in the mental health system was at least one person a week, and often more. There is a crisis in any situation where that many people die in a year due to strange or unsettling circumstances. Between self-harm and harm by others, being someone diagnosed with schizophrenia is immensely dangerous. It is too easy for something to happen. Schizophrenia has an enormously high rate of completed suicide, far outstripping the normal population in the country. This is the ultimate consequence of how our system lets people fall between the cracks.

Attending Community College with Schizophrenia

President Obama says that everybody in the United States should have at least one year of college prep in order to be ready for the workforce. After attending community college for over two years, from 2002-2005, I can attest to the need for skilled workers, as well as the fact that a university education makes your typical person more capable and mentally agile. As someone with a mental illness, I can also vouch for the role that college played in defining my capability and capacity to achieve and think of myself in a more global context.

Certainly, there were difficulties with enrolling and studying, even at the junior college level. I think a huge factor that served to hold me back from really tackling the difficult material was me: my self-esteem, and even how I conceived of myself, had been brutally affected by my dependence on the social service system. At the time that I restarted my studies, I had been on Social Security's disability program for seven years. Now, I refer to this as my forced sabbatical, or a life redirection (like you see on web pages – this is my own little technical joke).

That forced sabbatical meant that I only had a vague plan of college, graduate school, and work. I sure didn't have plans for dating and socializing. Apparently I missed the crib sheet explaining that a huge part of college life is making friends and learning how to be an adult. Thankfully, others would soon fill me in.

I met my first girlfriend in many, many years while in my freshman year – she was a feisty vegetarian who soon moved in with me. My family detested her, especially after she enforced her dietary choices on me. The fact that she had the standing ultimatum 'eat meat and I'll move out' didn't help smooth things over. That didn't last too long, and she moved in with her friend in a huff. To this day, I hold this lesson, amongst others, as my life guidepost for why dating is Hell.

There were plenty of people going to Lane Community – classes were packed, even then. Amidst budget cuts and spiraling unemployment, the local colleges were scooping up the disaffected; many people entered with hopes of staving off the recession, not necessarily graduating. There was a circle of younger students who treated the campus like a social scene. For these kids, classes were optional and parties mandatory. Abundant religious groups and tables filled with hard-core card players almost filled the cafeteria during most hours.

It was here that I leaned that as long as I was a little witty and mostly quiet, people would accept me without a second thought. Nobody ever asked me what medications I was taking or who my psychiatrist was. In college, the typical conversation revolved around easy teachers, hard classes, and managing the workload. Sadly, the numbers that one professor showed the workload was difficult for some. Only 40% of students completed their course of study at Lane Community, and fewer of these succeeded at the University of Oregon. It appeared that the cards were stacked against those who took the simple road via junior college.

I taught a Laurel Hill Center class, I worked as a peer mentor, and assisted people in enrolling at community colleges and universities. My numbers were even more abysmal than Lane's – while 40% of my students took tentative steps, nobody graduated from Lane during the year that I acted as a college mentor for people with mental illness. One huge reason was that people were comfortable making do with the bare minimum – disturbing the status quo meant losing housing, free food, and in the worst case, benefits. Benefits mean the difference between homelessness and an apartment, or medication vs. lack of medical care. When faced with the option to attend college and change their lives, most people in the social service system have been taught helplessness. Due to this, they pick a course of paralysis, and do nothing to change their life situation. To be fair, one cannot blame them for picking the safe path.

A Watchful Eye

Not many people with severe mental illness graduate from college. The number of enrollees with disabilities is rising, and has been increasing steadily over the last few decades. Whether this is attributable to better treatment, less stigma, or some other social element is difficult to say. From my personal experience teaching people with mental illness about how to access and succeed in college, the road is immensely difficult, and success is rare.

More people are attending college, and this includes people with schizophrenia and other forms of severe mental illnesses. When I was teaching a class at Laurel Hill Center about community college and mental health, the room was almost always packed with people eager to learn about ways to approach earning their college degree. There was a conundrum within this. Many of the people who had been in the system for decades had not earned their high school diploma, and a large proportion of the newly diagnosed people were suffering cognitive effects from the medication and illness. Thus, this group as a whole was entering with a handicap – the older from lack of knowledge, and the younger from lack of understanding.

The stigma regarding mental health meant that earlier than the 70s, people dropped out of high school or college once they were diagnosed, and seemed to have been given the implicit, unspoken message 'don't look back, you're not welcome in the halls of learning anymore.' I can only imagine being diagnosed in 1960, before the first effective antipsychotics and real treatments were developed, and being forced to struggle with my self-destructive mind for decades. So, in some ways the colleges were correct – for the majority of students with mania or psychotic thinking, higher academia was a goal beyond what many people with mental health issues could reasonably achieve. This was not always true then, and has been changing dramatically ever since the advent of psychotropic medication.

At the same time, after the 1970s, universities have been required to attempt to accommodate students with disabilities, as part of the Americans with Disabilities Act (ADA). While administrators may find this onerous, this legal mandate forced universities to cease discriminating against students with mental and physical disabilities, and also to make their campuses more welcoming and accessible to these groups. This kind of advocacy has been taken even farther by groups such as the National Alliance on Mental Illness (NAMI), which have established student-led groups on campuses around the USA that support and connect students with each other and the greater NAMI community as a whole.

Yet, the difficulty remains: people with disabilities have a lower graduation rate than non-disabled students, and enrollment within graduate school or doctoral programs is lower than the national average. So at a time where colleges are forcing themselves to enroll and accommodate students, the actual graduation rate for these groups is not on par with the national average. At Laurel Hill, I observed why people with mental illness may not graduate first-hand.

The people in my group had often suffered through the mental health system for years before starting to think about college. Often, while teaching the class, I would be interrupted by somebody having paranoia or delusions; one time, a student exclaimed 'I know what you're doing, and it isn't going to work,' and then stood up in a fury and stomped out of the room, screaming epithets. Often, people would just stand up and leave the classroom after

20 minutes, their attention exhausted long before the end of the 50 minute course I was teaching. If somebody could not handle 50 minute of friendly lecture, then college was going to be frustrating and difficult. Other times, people would nap in class or just not show up after scheduling themselves on my roster. When I followed up with these non-attendees, the answer was either 'I didn't feel like it,' or 'I was sleeping.' The combination of symptoms, apathy, and lethargy set the stage for failure before these people had ever set foot on campus.

Systemic Thoughts about Poverty

Mythology has various tales of the Hanged Man, Odin, or Jesus and 40 days in the wilderness –This is a metaphor for the journey of psychosis. Psychosis is a chance to peer inside the mind and examine what your deepest fears and desires are. In my introspective journey, I found that my passions and fears are often distinctly intertwined. For example, I feared being crazy and useless, and at the same time I had the deep dread of being independent and responsible. These are essentially flip sides of the same coin.

More so, there is a fear of being different that follows me. I was speaking with my wife over breakfast, and was able to voice this fear. I fear being a freak. Not just different, but a circus side-show. I can hear the barker now: "Look at the schizophrenic man work full time! Look at him pay his bills by himself! This is both amazing and unbelievable!" I think there would be a postcard rack or T-shirt stand outside the door. One out of a hundred people have schizophrenia, which puts me outside the bell curve already. The fear of being notably different propelled me towards the goal of almost every person with a psychotic past: I wanted to be normal. Hand me a white picket fence, 2.2 children, and a fuel-efficient car. Being normal is such a special feeling to me. My wife is always puzzled by the fact that one of my life goals is to be average.

The flip side is I want to be successful and noted – which is being different, but in a socially acceptable way. Why is being successful acceptable? Fame and power are more attractive than wealth, but any of these three accomplishments are far better than the prejudice of being labeled as mentally ill.

Somewhere along the line, I learned to be open about my diagnosis. It isn't out of fear of relapse, but I genuinely want people to be able to put a face to the word "schizophrenia." I have lost a lot of acquaintances due to this. I know pretty quickly when prejudice kicks in; sometimes a shift of the shoulders or a squinting of the eyes, but typically it is the sudden jerk away from where I'm sitting, like somebody just tugged on an invisible string or delivered an electric shock.

It seems that there is a critical threshold to reach when blending your professional life with the life of a mental health advocate. Will Hall, the founder of the Icarus Project (an organization devoted to recovery from mental illness while being medication-free) spoke of it in a blog – he doesn't know when to speak about his life as a mental health activist, but his mental health experiences are no secret. Right now, someone can find out my mental health status with a little digging. Google my name, and my past work with the National Alliance on Mental Illness comes up. At the same time, there are a few other unsavory work-related problems.

I worry about being the token mentally ill person (different circus, same show). Given the pay disparity that exists in our society, I am pretty sure there is a glass ceiling somewhere waiting for me to bump into it. And my pre-existing condition makes me about as uninsurable as someone with cancer or diabetes. When I think of these, I slip on my rose-tinted goggles and start pushing that boulder uphill.

That diagnosis of mental illness is crippling. The curious matter is that the agoraphobia, the social fear, the implosion of the self is part of the culture of mental illness. The people who work in the social service field are well intentioned. They are caregivers and providers, and take pride in their work. Yet the entire social fabric, from agency to individual, is designed to create failure. I avoided becoming one of those who fail, another number in the annual report, by luck. My family cared for me and set aside money for my education. Most of my friends accepted me, and stood by me in the initial years where I was reforming my identity. I had progress and opportunities to achieve, where most people are left behind. I am Malcolm Gladwell's outlier. I have grown jaded of hearing parents, teachers, and community members say, "You don't look mentally ill." Sometimes they couch it in "You look so good!" I guess it isn't quite correct to say, "You don't look impoverished and heavily medicated." I still don't have a good response to this comment. While I can acknowledge the sentiment, it is a backhanded compliment. Perhaps it is better to say nothing at all.

Especially critical was my self-concept. I never developed the concept of myself as mentally ill. My friends accepted me. In return for being 'odd' or 'strange,' I was given a place at the table. I was included during parties; I was invited on road-trips. All of this came at that critical point where I was re-discovering myself. Due to the fact that my social life was outside of the mental health/patient system, my thinking also existed outside the system. This was how I began to exit the system, several years after my grand entrance.

People conjure ideas of what it is like to be a number in the system. Whatever you can imagine does not quite touch on the truth. Being a patient in the system is boring – the medications make the barest effort difficult. Staying awake becomes a challenge; coffee was my best friend for years. The only people who drink more coffee than mental health patients are college students and truck drivers.

I have a confession: people do take advantage of the system. The truth is that anyone who does so in the vain hope of an easy life is selling themselves short. Many people whose parents were life-long recipients of social services grew up in the culture of poverty, a peculiar stratum of the chronically ill and working poor. That said, the majority of people I know needed the system at one point. The system is also the giver of critical medical care such as psychiatric services and case management. This is that dance of futility that I described already. People enter out of desperation, and stay out of necessity. They become adept at surviving with very little, and the first priority becomes resource protection. Thus the culture of poverty is instilled. This lifestyle is an issue for both sociology and education, and the very structure of it undermines every effort to escape.

Systemic Thoughts about Poverty, Part II

Sometimes I fear that I am dead already. A key to being able to achieve peace of mind is settling down with the idea that I may die. I faced death multiple times, and I think that nearly everyone with mental illness lives closer to death than most understand. Death seems to follow us. We who are in the mental health system die 25 years earlier than the average person in the USA. We have an incredibly high rate of suicide, and are often the victims of violence and homicide. Many mentally ill people are chronically homeless. Malnutrition or starvation frequently comes knocking at our door; many people depend on government surplus or food boxes comprised of outdated or donated food. Addictions haunt us, as many mentally ill people soothe themselves with alcohol or drugs.

This helped me to develop a blasé attitude towards death, but also a hypersensitivity that most don't have. I worry about dying, but I have sublimated this into a more socially salient fear: I worry about dying poor. To me, returning to the days where I survive by charity would be Sisyphean in scope. Like many Americans, I measure my self-worth by my paycheck. Or, to be accurate, I measure it by having a paycheck. Most people with mental illness do the same. Within our society, we're all trained that way, whether you are an airline pilot or a chronic patient. The difference is that one person is in charge of his or her life, and has direction (literally and metaphorically). The other is a lifelong passenger.

Finishing college put my earning potential outside the realm of most systemic dependents. Some people within my Eugene community wondered why I decided to leave the system, and not just volunteer or engage in activism. When it comes to the mental health system, there are things that evoke envy: Working half-time (but not full-time), earning more than minimum wage (but not too much more), and having any kind of side-benefit (except insurance). The reasons for this are complex and paradoxical. Working full-time means you will always earn too much, and lose your health and housing benefits. The same goes for having a higher wage. Having private insurance means you are responsible for co-pays, while with Medicaid, the government pays for everything. I understand this comfort with the status quo: Medications without insurance can run $1000 in a single month; one day in a psychiatric hospital can cost $1500. When I was in the system, I measured my assets by $1 increments. My total income was roughly $6000 a year. The poverty line is $16,000 a year.

Schizophrenia is a strange state, with the assumption made by society that people who have it exist in a vacuum, invisible and essentially non-existent. This isn't true; there is this certain microcosm that exists in the social service world for people with schizophrenia – and equally distinct realms for people who have schizophrenia and live outside of the social service network (typically due to the polar opposite scenarios of homelessness or extreme wealth.) There are written and unwritten hierarchies, values, and ways of life. All of these exist. People strive all their life to avoid ending up in the social service system, or at least that's the opinion that people have in our society.

Actually the truth of it is there are quite a few people who would love to be in the service system because it provides a kind of safety net. Being enmeshed in the safety net is not the most effective thing for having a successful life. There is difficulty in living in that kind of impoverished state. I lived there for years. Thinking about it brings up the past, thinking about all those lives that I was part of. These people are moored in the system but often invisible, waiting for someone to notice them. That's what it's like, being in the social service system – there is a sense of quiet desperation.

I look at myself now, having a Master's degree, having graduated from college, being married to Jessica, my wonderful wife, and living in Philadelphia. This world seems so sunny and bright. It is so far removed from the world of social services and disabilities that my life truly seems to have a split right down the middle: before and after recovery. In many ways, the past is a shadow – it is always present with me, but never speaks.

Extreme and abject poverty wait beyond the gates of the social service system, yet many people accuse people with mental illness of being lazy or useless to society. Give us health care, is my argument to the skeptics. Assure a halfway decent support network, and medical care, and we will leave the system in droves. And remember that no one chooses to suffer from mental illness, any more than people choose to have cancer or multiple sclerosis.

Social Animals

My own college path had its own set of challenges. I found that making friends in college is easy. But making friends in college and successfully graduating is a step harder. After I enrolled in community college for the second time, my social network expanded well beyond the limited fabric of Eugene's local mental health system. Even more importantly, I began dating and having romantic relationships once again; this was a huge step, as I had thought that I would be alone for my lifetime. My approach to romance was greatly different than it had been in high school, which was the last time I had had a relationship. Over the years since my initial diagnosis, I had the chance to mature in many ways, stepping back from the befuddlement that comes with youth. Amidst all this, I was also forced to swiftly and accurately judge potential friends and partners for prejudice against schizophrenia. Without a doubt, this reduced my dating pool – I was forced to swiftly locate people who did not seem to discriminate against others. If my first impression indicated bias or contempt for others, I became wary and guarded, and in some ways hyper vigilant.

At Lane Community College, my friends stretched from older students retraining after career implosions, to freshman who had graduated from high school merely months before. The difference in dedication seemed directly proportional to age and desperation, as the older students had much more on the line – often, if they didn't get good enough grades, there was no second option. Also, the older, non-traditional students often had families, children, and people depending on them. If the younger students had these burdens and responsibilities, I'm unaware of it. One nickname for the younger group was the 'babysitter's club', as they often skipped class in order to play cards and hang out in the cafeteria. In contrast, the older students fled to the library immediately after class was out, determined to grasp concepts and ideas that they often had never encountered before.

Upon my graduation from community college, I enrolled at the University of Oregon, where the caliber of student and academic rigor was much greater. Here I would continue to hide my identity as somebody with schizophrenia, determined to let this aspect of my life fade into the background so that I could reinvent myself as an erudite scholar and potential graduate student.

Graduate school was even within my grasp. After the University of Oregon, I finished my first master's at Drexel University in library and information science, and then I re-enrolled in a second master's program in information systems. My goal was to push myself as far as I could go academically and professionally. My understanding was that the more education I obtained, the more employable I would become, and the further from failure I would be. In the end, my efforts, combined with a healthy dose of luck, paid off and earned my place as a data analyst at the University of Pennsylvania Medical System, and later led to working as a data scientist for Kaiser Permanente, wherein I developed predictive models and worked on large data analytics projects.

Friendships and Romance With Schizophrenia

Relationships are hard work – anybody who tells you otherwise has an agenda. They require compromise and negotiation, patience, and the ability to understand things from another person's perspective. Sure, you can get by not having one or two of these skills. But if you, or your partner, are unwilling or unable to learn any of these basic social skills, watch out – you just boarded the Rollercoaster to Hell.

Take what I just said, tone it down a notch or two, and you have the same basic formula for making, keeping, and losing friends. Typically, keeping friends requires a little less work – unless they are the intensely needy kind that you would probably be better without. When your friendship with somebody requires more work than your romantic and/or intimate partnership, you have a powder keg waiting for the spark. Explosions may or may not immediately happen, but if the setting becomes primed, the charge will blow.

I dated quite a bit in those years between my first diagnosis and when I met my future wife, Jessica. Part of my non-failure as a partner stemmed from my experiences within the mental health system, and being patient – with me, with my partner, and also the relationship as well. Good relationships need tending, and then they will blossom. Even an excellent marriage will wither if neglected long enough – attention and time is the key to success. Via both first-hand and second-hand experiences, I had the chance to learn what worked well, and what led to misery. Having schizophrenia ended up being the least of my worries, because the dating experience is a cesspool of chaos for everybody. Whenever one of my friends tells me that they are beginning to date, I wish them well – and wince on the inside.

For instance, I dated a woman – she was a little punky, and very creative. She took a backpack and turned it into a replica of a Muppet – huge fabric teeth surrounded the zipper, and bubble eyes stuck out of the top. For my birthday, she knitted a hat that looked like a panda bear – this was far before any retailer thought to do this. She was unique.

Then she dumped me to date a high-school friend. Amongst her many apologies was one tidbit that I filed away in my consciousness – she said this: 'My dad had a head injury, and I saw how it affected my mom; I just couldn't see myself in a long-term relationship with you, because the same kind of thing could happen to us.' I don't recall how often I have been compared to people with traumatic brain injury, but I can reassure you it isn't often. We had dated about a year, and I had been thinking that things were going along pretty well. It is experiences like this that cause me to shiver with fear for my dating friends – the potential for heartbreak and confusion is vast, like a sea of stars. Even though there is a perfect star out there waiting for everybody, it is too easy to get moored in the wrong place. This woman was an example of that, but it wasn't the first time that I had been spurned or refused due to my past history of psychosis.

I'm sorry that I sound bitter when talking about this. Forming relationships is quite challenging when you live with chronic, low-grade paranoia about the people around you. After being rebuked and/or mocked for having a chronic health condition, it is easy to become sensitive and withdraw. Too often, I was either openly insulted or isolated due to my illness.

There was one group of people that I had been forming close friendships with. We went to coffee shops and idled the time, watched movies together, and had a social life of sorts – until I stumbled into a conversation that went like this:

'Everybody with mental illness is the victim of childhood sexual trauma,' one man exclaimed proudly.

'How did you reach that conclusion?' I asked, bewildered.

'I learned it in college. My professor taught us about this. She was a great teacher, and I did really well in her class. I even graduated with honors, double-major in psychology and sociology!' He grinned his toothy grin, which he was well known for. That smile was why his girlfriend ended up marrying him, I am pretty sure. Never before had I wanted to slap the smile off his foolish face.

Now keep in mind that I was sitting at a table, in a coffee shop, surrounded by four people who I was socially engaged with. I figured it was a 'go big or go home' kind of moment, so I burst his bubble.

'You know, I have schizophrenia, and I was never sexually abused.' And my eyes looked at all of them, one after another. From the moment I looked at the first person, I knew that my social circle had just contracted by four people – these people's prejudices and self-righteous pseudo-knowledge had conquered the day.

I was right about that, too – after all, I had been telling people about my mental illness for over 12 years. The art of disclosure was pretty well tuned for me. People either fell into two categories: open and curious, or politely distant. The former would remain my friends, and the latter would find a reason to distance themselves from me. This is how my world went: after I told somebody, I had about a 25% chance they would remain a friend. It was a risky position for me to take. Writing this memoir is an even greater risk: socially, professionally, and personally.

Shortly after I told this group of people about my diagnosis, somebody needed to get home and take care of the laundry. Another person seconded that. It was nice that they offered me a ride home, but there was no hug afterwards as I got out of the car like there usually was. In the minds of others, psychosis is contagious, or dangerous. After a few weeks, I noticed that I had been unfriended on the social networks. Of course I stopped receiving invitations to do anything social – that was instantaneous. Schizophrenia is lonely, and I am well acquainted with being alone.

She Married Somebody Difficult

It takes a brave and strong woman to marry a man with schizophrenia. In case that isn't broad enough, let's stretch this concept out: it takes a strong person to marry somebody with mental illness. Period. If the difficulty of the illness doesn't eventually interfere, then the stigma and societal prejudice will be an ever-present facet of the partnership.

My wife is an thread throughout all of the story that I've shared. It should be made clear that she doesn't share my belief in the magical nature of things. As a matter of fact, she often questions the reality of my experiences, and is convinced that I was merely highly delusional during most of the fantastical events I endured. As a psychologist, her training is focused around cognitive behavioral therapy for psychosis, a modality of therapy much more common in the United Kingom than the United States. Her expertise and affectionate understanding of my peculiar world-view has led to some intriguing conversations – about what the moral obligation is for parents if the family has a history of mental illness, about the social service system and ways to teach consumer empowerment, and about the very nature of psychosis itself. I'm convinced they she'll never believe in anything magical or extra-numinous; I don't think her highly logical kind and years of rigorous training will allow her to wander down that path. Hence, she acts as a bulwark against my flights of fancy, which all too often have nearly led me into the dark chasms where my psychosis attempts to go. Without her, I would truly be lost in a sea of fog, or left to wander alone in this planet of sand.

We met in Eugene. I remember meeting her and having an instant spark; I also recall that I panicked that evening and took a double dose of my antipsychotic medication, fearing that I'd appear weird otherwise. Little did I know that Jessica had spent years in Boston as a live-in transitional housing counselor, and that she was perfectly at home with people whom most others would immediately label 'nuts', 'crazy', of 'dangerous'. To her, I am a person first; schizophrenic doesn't even make the top 5 descriptive words she uses when describing me.

Just as importantly, my mental illness isn't a cop-out. At no point can I just play the 'mental illness' card and call my efforts good. She pushes me to excel in numerous ways (and pulls double duty keeping my ego in check). Not a simple task when your husband is prone to delusions of grandeur (perhaps more like wishful thinking, nowadays). She perseveres throughout all of her work, and I can attest to her intelligence and dedication to our daughter and our family, which now stretches from Hawaii to the East Coast.

How I Met Your Mother: The Mental Health Version

I met Jessica, my wife, at an Italian bistro near campus. That's not really quite true: I met her online, at OKCupid.com, where I promptly panicked and wrote her a missive aptly titled 'We can be friends, but we can never date.' A few years later we were married in Hawaii at Lanikuhonua, a nature preserve and lush ocean-side park.

My fear originated in my loneliness. When you have given yourself the 'it's OK to be alone' speech hundreds of times, you get acquainted with the concept of being single, just like you learn to assimilate the subtler self-definition of 'broken'. Society will not hesitate before labeling somebody as defective or worth less than others. Even with years of recovery under my belt, my life still demands that I pause and evaluate my success and self-worth.

Jessica obviously saw value in my life and my experiences. Other people that I had dated missed out on the narrative of my schizophrenia, deeming it 'behind me' or 'just a troublesome phase of my life'. Jessica was curious and accepting. She believed in me as a person, and knew that my previous life was just as precious as any other part of my life, not something to wall off and forget about.

I've been blessed with a number of people in my life that accepted my history and peculiarities with grace. When necessary, these people rose to the challenge of helping me with my psychosis. Jessica is foremost of these people whom have been instrumental in helping my life transition from imbalanced to balanced, disoriented to clear-sighted, and unwelcomed to loved.

Children and Family: Living with the Black Dog

We have two black dogs. They live in Hawaii, with Jessica's parents. Both dogs are well treated, even spoiled – the fact that Jessica's parents have watched both dogs for over two years is a measure of the love that her parents have for us. While we migrate from place to place (moving from Hawaii to Philadelphia, and then to the Willamette Valley in Oregon, and who knows where afterwards), the dogs dutifully wait for us like friendly shadows. They bide their time and are joyous when we return to Oah'u and visit them.

Part of the joy and burden of owning pets is that they require attention. Unlike houseplants, an animal necessitates feeding and providing. You cannot just put your pet out on the patio or it becomes feral and sullen, or worse. The worst dogs aren't the dogs that aren't kept, but the dogs that are ill kept. The same goes for caring for the health of a family.

Mentally, physically, and spiritually, a family demands diligence and love. My wife, Jessica, allows me to sometimes become lax with the affection and attention, but at the end of the day it is my family that stands by me. I take care of them, and they provide a center for peace and stability in my sometimes whirlwind life. Jessica and I have a daughter, Liv, whom was born recently. In some ways, I ponder how we as parents will care for Liv's black dogs when the time comes.

Liv's dogs are likely to be distinctly different from the burdensome dogs that Jessica and I raised from puppies. Sometimes I wonder whether she'll have the same shadowy hound follow her life that follows mine. My schizophrenia trails me like a loyal canine, always at my side. It waits to leap into action, frolic into madness, and bring my world crashing to a halt. My medications are the key to keeping my dog well heeled. Through her diligence and hard work, Jessica has helped me train my mind to better control the psychotic episodes when they emerge. Her compassion and thoughtfulness, as well as acceptance, has been critical to my recovery. For everyone whom recovers, there is at least one person who believes in that person, fully, whole-heartedly. Jessica believes in my ability to heal and achieve my potential. She has taught me to be my own physician, for as the saying goes: 'Physician, heal thyself.'

Liv may be forced to face off against her shadow. These are the kinds of things that we don't know – we cannot, as a species, see the future of where we are going. The best we can approximate is an educated guess. My guess would be predicated on probability: Liv is not likely to develop psychosis or schizophrenia, but her slim chance is greater than most people's risk. Hereditary studies show that there is a 10% chance for a direct descendant to develop the illness, which was definitely part of Jessica and my discussion when Liv arrived. It is one thing to say '1 out of 10 is a chance we can take', and another thing to hold your newborn baby daughter and think the same thought.

Overall, there is a grand bargain with life that we make: in return for opportunity, we barter that we'll be given risks, unacceptable and grave. This is the way that life churns within the six realms of *samsara*: all life has an origin in challenge. Yet, at the same time, I sometimes find myself praying in the smallest hours of the night that the world knows more peace, that there is less storm and thunder. I wish that Liv's childhood, especially, and adulthood, can be free from the burdens of this era, and that the weight of the next hundred years is far lighter than the shackles of the prior century.

The Caul

My family hails from Scotland, mostly. We have a bit of Native American in us; Cherokee and Mohawk Apache, or so the speculation goes. Another part of our lineage comes from Ireland, but mostly Scotch-Irish. If you ask my sister, we also have a large Teutonic/German genetic component, which may explain my persuasion for runes and ancient myth. Anyway you look at the family heritage, the Scottish part of the family is strong and present.

The Scottish have incorporated many elements into their culture, little and big, that now play a part in my daily life. For instance, there is the cultural belief in the Little People. I'm not referencing Darby O'Gill and his merry band of pranksters. The Faerie, or Fair Ones, are deeply embedded in the landscape and society of the United Kingdom. When I looked for knowledge about my excursion into the Otherlands, the lore and myths of England and Scotland proved the deepest pool.

These myths are where I learned all kinds of things: the Fey fear the touch of cold iron, which dispels their powers; mentioning the name of Jesus Christ out loud also temporary sends them hither. They won't enter churches, and they disdain the sound of church bells, which are painful. They delight in trickery and deceit; to the Fair Ones, anyone, anywhere, can be fair game to a mischievous prank. And the curses they level upon dimwitted trespassers are horrifying and torturous.

Other scraps of wisdom slowly drifted my ways, gathered over the years after my forays into the forest. Every few months, I would search out books or articles about magic and mystery. The pinnacle of my search was found in two thin manuscripts. These dated from the early 1800s. I read quite a few books about Faerie magic and sorcery before I realized that most of these authors made a living by penning these books for hopeful dreamers. After that, I turned to older books and folktales; these books proved much more useful.

One specific work was especially useful: a priest wrote it in the late 1800s, as he ministered to the people of the Highlands. This priest wrote extensively about the Sight of the Scottish folk. A huge portion of the Gift of the Sight relates to the Fey and the Otherlands. Not everyone with the Sight relates to magic in the same way, but for all people with at least a glimmer of the Gift, strange things can and would happen. Sometimes people could see the future, getting a peek of what was to come in a dream or daytime vision. Others could tell when somebody's end was near, even when such a thing seemed distant or unlikely. A third common Gift was being able to see the Faerie and interact with them as if they were present, here and now. Tied into all of this was the thread of the land that held the Gifted tight to the Otherworld.

When somebody with the Sight had it too bad, wrote the priest, it was misery. Rarely did any good come from these powers. As a matter of fact, the priest was determined to prove that the Sight was an inherently natural function, instead of a supernatural or evil power granted by the Devil. Ah, such was the thinking of the 1800s: metaphysical and paranormal studies had yet to be discarded in favor of hard science. Thus, this serious entreaty into Scottish folklore and Otherworldly gifts was both well written and studiously documented in the methods of the era.

Poignantly, there was one remedy for a family member whose Sight proved too much to bear. The answer was strangely paradoxical – send them abroad, never to return to Scotland. If the Gift was too vast and unsettling, daughters and sons would relocate to a different country entirely – this seemed to be effective in quelling the Gift. Apparently, the Sight is highly tied to the land of origin. I know that once I left the Northwest to move to Hawaii and then Pennsylvania, my symptoms receded to a non-existent level (I continued taking my medications as a prophylactic measure), but returning to Oregon for a single day caused my old patterns to begin to re-emerge.

Another story about the Fey and Scotland deals with the birthing caul. A caul is the amniotic sac, which sometimes covers a baby's face when they are born. This is very, very rare; such children are considered to be strong with the Sight. Another myth goes that caul-born children have been touched by the Fair Ones, or even replaced at birth by a Faerie seeking entrance into the world of Man. Whatever the truth to the caul birth stories, it is somehow intertwined with my own tale: my mother was born with a caul.

Road Echoes

We came around the curve in the road, the purple heather hills sprawling out like crinkled paper as far as the eye could stretch itself – the horizon wasn't far enough for the Scottish Highland hills to reach. Pulling over to the side of the road, I hopped out of the driver's side door and breathed in the crisp air.

I heard the car's door shut behind me, and Jessica also began walking around the parking lot. We were deep on the northern shore of the Scottish Highlands. About all we could see on any direction was the before-mentioned purple heather, sheep, and Highland cows, a distinctive, shaggy, huge-horned beast that was a favorite local livestock. Between each low-slung mountain was a valley, and every valley had a loch at one end, where the earth dipped down into the lowest point. The rain was frequent and heavy, even in the heart of summer. Brisk, constant winds stripped the leaves from the trees and rustled the flowers. Every few hours, the light would pierce the clouded sky in what Jessica had taken to calling 'Jesus light'. This was when a handful of sunbeams would breach the clouds and launch towards the earth. It was for all intents the same lighting as on those infamous office motivational posters from the mid-1990s – the difference was that we were in Scotland, seeing it first-hand, on our honeymoon.

I was plagued by feverish dreams since arriving in Edinburgh. I kept having mental images of things moving between invisible spaces, like a flicker of shadow in mannish form. The ravens, those huge, black crow-cousins, seemed to be stalking me. A few times I swore that I saw things directly, like gnarly goblins hiding in an alley, or a man wrapped in a black, tattered coat that stood within an archway and watched Jessica and I pass, one

129

finger raised to his lips as a warning. The United Kingdom was a tough place for me to be. The Sight never turned off the entire trip, not fully, and it continuously seethed under my eyes and burned like a fire in my head. There was fear and anxiety, but little rest to be had.

At one particular road stop, somewhere along a stretch of two-lane road running 40 kilometers south of the Scottish coast, we found a fascinating sight. We tumbled down the hillside, curious enough to brave the bog below. At the base of the hill was a road, broken like cobblestone. One end of this old road ran straight into a large, lush forest about a mile away. These trees stretched along the flank of the Scottish hillside, and were mostly coniferous, pine-type woods. The other end of the road ran into a loch. Not alongside, but directly into and through the loch. As soon as my feet stepped out of the waterlogged bog and onto the roadway, I knew I was in danger. My internal alarm went off, alerting me that something had gone awry. The trap was sprung. I didn't know how long this snare had lain in wait for someone like me, but within a moment I felt the lasso close around my mind.

'Come'. The wind spoke to me. 'Come into the trees. We are waiting for you.' I turned and started down the road, oblivious to Jessica, who was standing and staring at me, confused.

'Babe!' Jessica said. 'Babe? Will? What's wrong? Where are you going?' She looked at me, perhaps a bit worried. At the very least, she was obviously bewildered.

'Let's go into the woods, Jess. It's so weird, let's go look at the other end of this road.' Stumbling over my words, I tried to sound excited. Instead, I could hear panic within my words.

'No, let's get out of here. This is creepy all of a sudden.'
She turned to climb up the hillside towards the Vauxhall
two-door economy car we were touring the countryside in.

I tried arguing a bit, but this time the curse didn't have
time to cinch shut around me before I escaped. As I
reached the top of the bank and looked back towards the
mysterious road, the loch, and the woods, the sun seemed
the crawl behind the clouds. At the same time, a raven that
had been perched on a rock nearby launched itself into the
sky, cawing madly. It dove towards the woods. A raucous
sound erupted from the woods, and an unkindness of
black birds flew out to meet our spy. My heart sunk, and it
was then that I knew I could never settle in the United
Kingdom – this land was hostile to me, and I was uneasy
with the trees and animals. They seemed different then the
carefree spirits of the Northwest.

In My Mind

Even now, on a daily basis, I sometimes experience moments of anxiety or terror, or slip into a bit of a fugue state where I imagine otherworldly events occurring around me. For example, I may be sitting in a coffee shop and suddenly have the conviction that the person at the table next to me is a vampire or Faerie being. Another common thought is that a co-worker is trying to mentally control me with latent psychic powers, or that I am trapped in a mental battle with a fellow student or somebody that I have had a disagreement with. The key to all of these mental illusions is that there is a component of conflict and stress that plays out.

Many people manifest stress by eating unhealthily or drinking. But I manifest stress by playing out conflict in the arena of my imagination; in this, there is nothing new. Many people ruminate over their life, dwelling over failed chances or things that could have gone better. Due to my vivid imagination, I take this one step farther: in my mind's eye, I play out cosmic events like a galactic theater, doing battle for good. It is ironic that at the same time I am mentally roughing up the people around me, part of my mind thinks that it is defending itself from attackers, or assisting to defeat evil, or otherwise championing some far-flung, noble cause. Thankfully, after reading Thich Nhat Hahn and the Dalai Lama, I have concluded that everybody in the world has erroneous, crazy messages playing through their head all the time.

Thoughts can be like a wagon, and they can wear grooves in the tracks of the mind— and then later thoughts follow those grooves, repeating behaviors, actions, and beliefs. When I had my psychotic break, apparently my mind churned the road's mud pretty deep, and left some tracks that are almost impossible for my mind not to follow. This is where my medication comes in, as it helps to free me from compulsions and grandiose ideas. It is a huge warning sign when my mind cannot diverge from the patterns that it formed on my 18th birthday. It took me over a decade to form the level of adeptness and clarity of thought that is required to hold my mind from getting stuck in the mire of my psychotic thought patterns – when I first fell ill, paranoia and warrantless suspicions destroyed most of my friendships. Only after years of introspection have I realized that I have a high level of latent mistrust, which is so often kindled into outright paranoid thoughts. Thanks to Buddhist teachings, I realized that the goal isn't perfect lucidity, but clarity and functionality. Buddhism helped me realize that the core of paranoid is anxiety and fear, and ultimately a lack of perceived control over the world. Once I was able to begin solving this dilemma, my paranoia simmered down to a low boil, rather than a raging kettle of panic.

It is amazing to think of what the person next to you could be imagining while you are drinking coffee. Everybody has a world within the mind, a world all their own. The key is that nobody can see within it, and it exists only within the confines of self-consciousness. Within my mind is a universe of conflict and bliss that mirrors the external world I live in; I think that this is true for everybody. My friends used to have a saying, before we all begin selling out and becoming lawyers and professionals: 'Subvert the Dominant Paradigm.' My subconscious thinking warps and twists reality on a constant ongoing basis – but only in a purely subjective manner.

While my internal world is askew, twirling like a Mobius strip into fantastical worlds, my outside world is consistent with everybody else's perceptions. As Buddhism teaches, the mind is a monkey at play in the forest; it always seeks to entertain and spin tales. It is always grasping at thoughts, jumping, and chattering; when it gets angry, it throws coconuts.

Sum

Being diagnosed with schizophrenia does not signal the end of life; the majority of people recover over a 30-year span, successfully stopping medications and returning to the world that they left behind during their psychotic episode. Over nearly twenty years, I traveled from being outcast on the fringes of society and circled back into the folds of a fully involved life. From isolation and paranoia, I spiraled out into the chasms of psychosis, and over a decade my life returned to normal. People with a mental health history can live a vibrant, full life with children, marriage, work, school, and all the trappings and obligations that society asks of its members.

Harboring a mental illness means being extra-careful and diligent. Mindfulness and self-awareness lead to insights into the human condition of living with a chronic health condition. Part of recovery is moving past that self-definition of 'sickly' and replacing it with a self-conceptualization that revolves around strength and self-acceptance. Indeed, being able to look at myself in the mirror was and is crucial towards overcoming my shadow, that temperamental and trickery part of my being that seeks to undo my accomplishments.

Yet, there is that small voice within all of us, the duality of the angel and devil that gives unwanted advice and steers our actions for right or wrong. Knowing how to identify myself, that voice that I call me, from the myriad of thoughts, wants, and desires within my conscious mind has led me to freedom from the social service system and allowed me to resume the life that I had left behind on my 18th birthday. From a magical beginning, I've proudly entered the world of the mundane, and this is where I strive to be. Being normal is an achievement, and one that I am happy with.

For anyone whom has a family member with schizophrenia, or those people given the life burden of hearing voices and dealing with confusion and psychosis, I would give you the heart-felt message: It gets better. Over time, learning to live with psychosis and the problems and conundrums that the illness causes will give way to knowledge – it may not happen immediately, and can move with the speed of molasses, but one drop at a time change will occur within the internal world of schizophrenia. This isn't just true for me, but I can firmly say that recovery is possible for anyone. It may not come in the form of a pill bottle, but can instead arrive in the voices of a friend, a loved one, or even yourself. What people with schizophrenia need to hear, more than anything else, are the words 'I believe in you. You'll get better.'

To which I say, to those reading this whose lives have been impacted by mental illness: 'I do believe in you, and you will indeed get better.' Carry this with you, and remember.

ABOUT THE AUTHOR

William Brundage works as a 1) father, 2) husband, and 3) data scientist. In his spare time he creates works of fiction and graphic novels revolving around mental health and spirituality, and the often strange juxtaposition of the two worlds. He is a resident of his beloved Pacific Northwest.

www.ingramcontent.com/pod-product-compliance
Lightning Source LLC
Chambersburg PA
CBHW051318170526
45166CB00002B/588